Epigenetics

Edited by Rosaria Meccariello

Published in London, United Kingdom

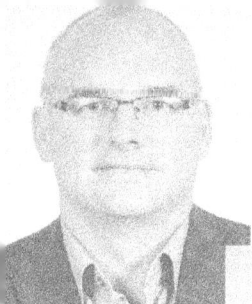
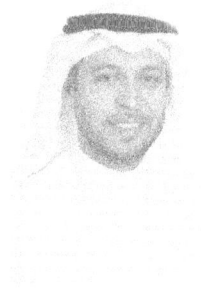
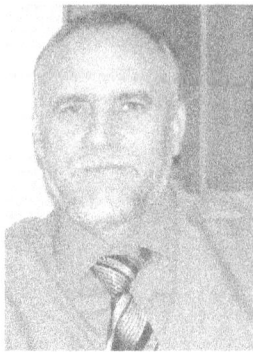
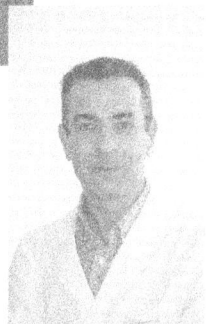
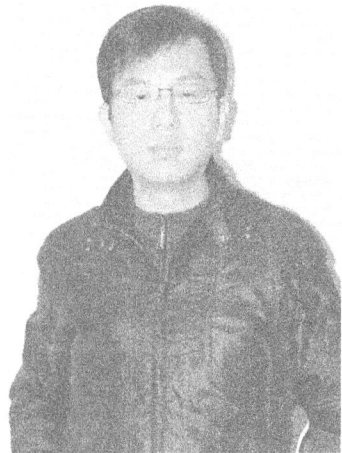
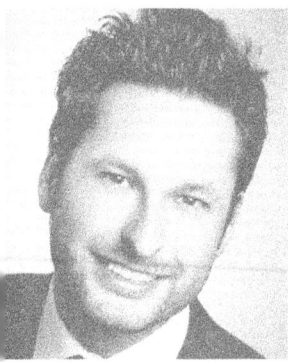
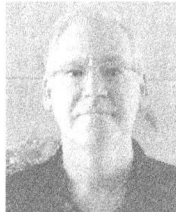

IntechOpen

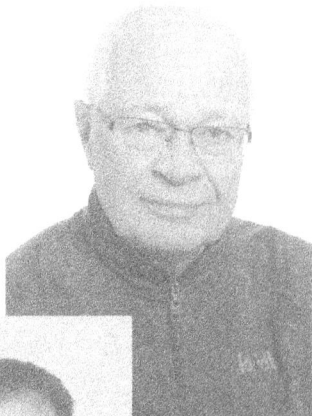
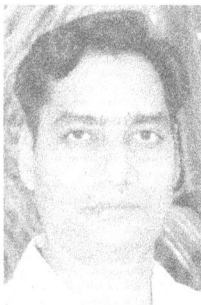
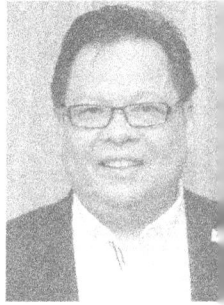
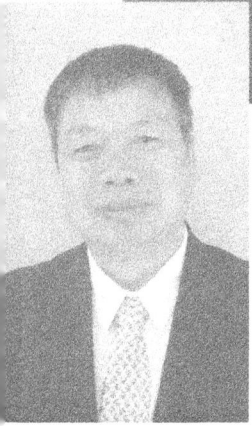
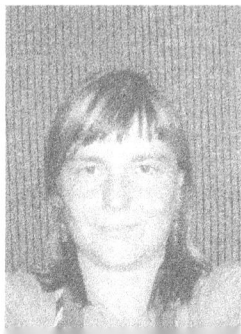
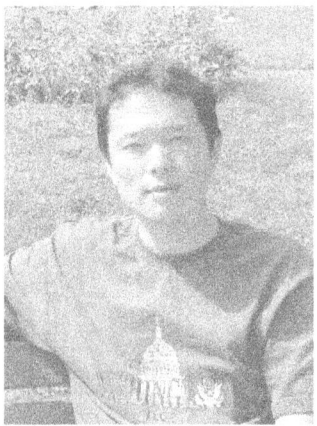

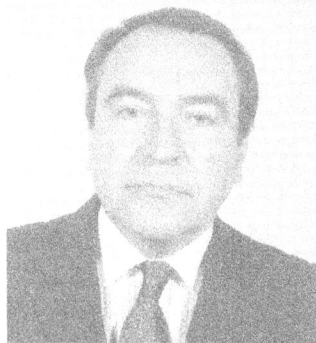

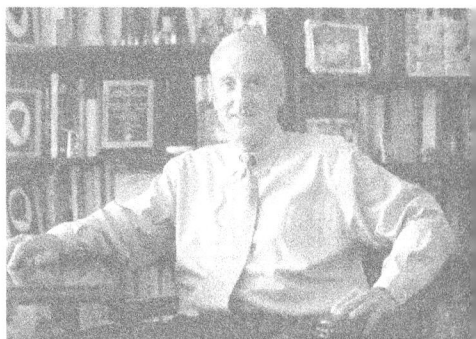

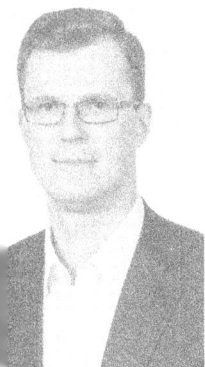

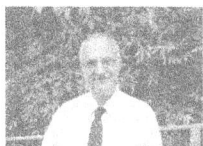

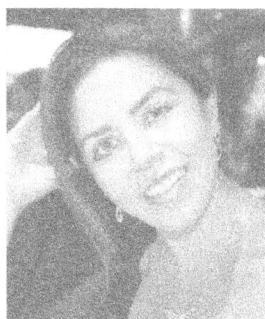

Supporting open minds since 2005

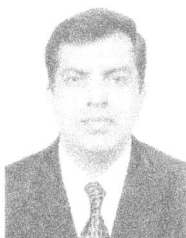

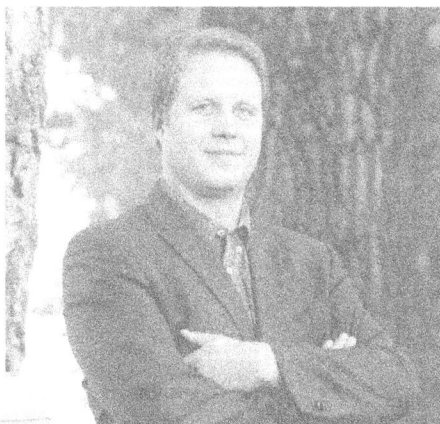

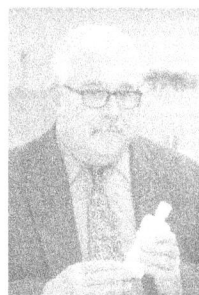

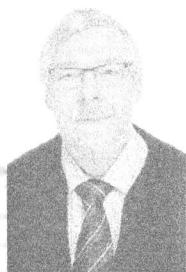

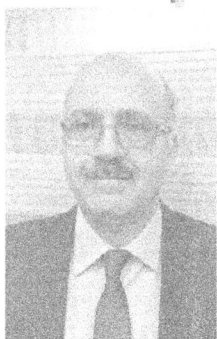

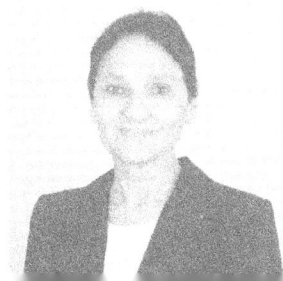

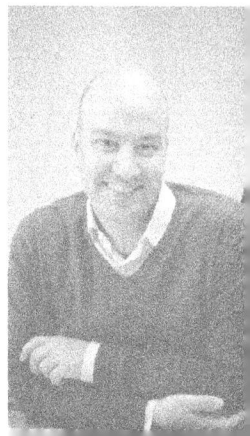

Epigenetics
http://dx.doi.org/10.5772/intechopen.77825
Edited by Rosaria Meccariello

Contributors
Apiwat Mutirangura, Tiago Fernandes, João Lucas Penteado Gomes, Ursula Paula Renó Soci, Edilamar
Menezes De Oliveira, Gabriel Cardial Tobias, Garima Singroha, Pradeep Sharma, Abed Elsalam Zubidat,
Abraham Haim, Sinam Boynao, Rosaria Meccariello

Notice
Statements and opinions expressed in the chapters are these of the individual contributors and not
necessarily those of the editors or publisher. No responsibility is accepted for the accuracy of
information contained in the published chapters. The publisher assumes no responsibility for any
damage or injury to persons or property arising out of the use of any materials, instructions, methods
or ideas contained in the book.

First published in London, United Kingdom, 2019 by IntechOpen
IntechOpen is the global imprint of INTECHOPEN LIMITED, registered in England and Wales,
registration number: 11086078, The Shard, 25th floor, 32 London Bridge Street
London, SE19SG – United Kingdom
Printed in Croatia

British Library Cataloguing-in-Publication Data
A catalogue record for this book is available from the British Library

Additional hard and PDF copies can be obtained from orders@intechopen.com

Epigenetics
Edited by Rosaria Meccariello
p. cm.
Print ISBN 978-1-78984-087-2
Online ISBN 978-1-78984-088-9
eBook (PDF) ISBN 978-1-83881-970-5

We are IntechOpen,
the world's leading publisher of
Open Access books
Built by scientists, for scientists

4,300+
Open access books available

116,000+
International authors and editors

125M+
Downloads

Our authors are among the

151
Countries delivered to

Top 1%
most cited scientists

12.2%
Contributors from top 500 universities

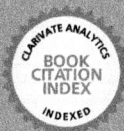

Interested in publishing with us?
Contact book.department@intechopen.com

Numbers displayed above are based on latest data collected.
For more information visit www.intechopen.com

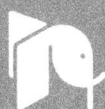

Meet the editor

Dr. Rosaria Meccariello obtained a degree in Biological Sciences from the University of Naples Federico II, Italy, and a PhD in Comparative Endocrinology from the University of Padova, Italy. Currently, she is Associate Professor of Biology at the Department of Movement and Wellness Sciences at the University of Naples "Parthenope," Italy. She has published more than 130 papers in peer-reviewed international journals, books, proceedings and abstract books. She has experience as a reviewer for international journals and has served as an editor for scientific books, special issues and e-books. Dr. Meccariello is an expert in biology of reproduction, spermatogenesis, the hypothalamus-pituitary-gonad axis, central and local activity of GnRH, endocannabinoid and kisspeptin systems, and epigenetics.

Contents

Preface

Epigenetic changes are heritable and reversible modifications that significantly affect gene expression without any change in DNA sequence. Epigenetic mechanisms include DNA methylation, imprinting, chromatin remodelling via histone modifications, and the production of specific non-coding RNA. The epigenetic signature is remodelled during the lifespan as a direct consequence of both environment and lifestyle. Therefore, health or disease status strongly depends on epigenetic marks. In addition, the epigenetic signature of gametes and parental experience may cause transgenerational epigenetic inheritance, thus affecting offspring health. Lastly, emerging evidence reveals that epigenetic marks, and in particular circulating non-coding RNAs, represent upcoming biomarkers for the prevention, diagnosis and treatment of diseases.

This book summarizes the current knowledge in the field of epigenetics in five chapters. Chapter 1 provides a brief introduction to epigenetics and is followed by a study on epigenetics in plants (Chapter 2) and three chapters concerning epigenetics in health and disease: cancer (Chapter 3), the photoperiodic system (Chapter 4) and aging (Chapter 5).

Chapter 2 by Drs. Singroha and Sharma describes the epigenetic regulation of the plant genome, focusing on the epigenetic modifications in plants under abiotic stress.

Environmental factors and lifestyle both affect epigenetic marks. Thus, Chapter 3 by Dr. Tobias et al. analyses the role of microRNAs in cancer and cachexia, pointing out the possible contribution of physical activity to tumor regression.

Chapter 4 by Dr. Haim et al. describes the consequences of artificial light at night and the links between chasing darkness away and epigenetic modifications.

Lastly, Chapter 5 by Dr. Mutirangura presents an interesting hypothesis for aging based on genome-wide hypomethylation. Such a condition may cause genomic instability and aging-associated disease phenotypes, thus explaining how the DNA of elderly people is prone to damage.

Taken together, the chapters in this book target a wide audience of basic and clinical scientists, teachers and students interested in gaining a better understanding of epigenetics.

Rosaria Meccariello
University of Naples Parthenope,
Italy

Chapter 1

Introductory Chapter: Epigenetics in Summary

Rosaria Meccariello

1. Definition

In 1940 the developmental biologist Conrad H. Waddington firstly used the term "epigenetics" to describe "*the interaction of genes with their environment, which bring the phenotype into being*" [1]. Two years later, Conrad Waddington pointed out that "*It is possible that an adaptive response can be fixed without waiting for the occurrence of a mutation*" [2]. Thus, epigenetic modifications are heritable and reversible modifications that significantly affect gene expression without any change in the nucleotide sequence of DNA [3].

2. Molecular mechanisms

Classically, epigenetic mechanisms include (i) the methylation of DNA, (ii) the imprinting, (iii) the remodeling of chromatin, and (iv) the production of noncoding RNA (ncRNA) [4, 5].

The methylation of DNA usually occurs at the 5-position of DNA cytosine (5mC) in the CpG islands located within the promoter region of specific genes; such a modification inhibits both the binding of transcription factors to DNA and affects the recruitment of proteins involved in chromatin remodeling [6, 7], thus causing gene silencing.

Genomic imprinting is a DNA methylation-dependent phenomenon, occurring during embryogenesis; it causes genes to be expressed from a parent of origin-specific manner [8] and specifically interests at some genetic loci.

Nuclear DNA is structured in chromatin, an instructive DNA scaffold that can respond to external cues regulating DNA activity, composed of histone and nonhistone proteins [9]. Euchromatin, which is the transcriptionally active region of the DNA, represents the loosely folded part of the chromatin; heterochromatin, which is a transcriptionally poorly active region of the DNA, represents the tightly folded part of the chromatin [10]. Therefore, the transcription rate of genes is strongly affected by dynamic chromatin remodeling. In this respect, posttranslational modifications of histone tails like methylation and acetylation play critical roles, by affecting either the affinity of transcriptional factors for gene promoter region or the recruitment to chromatin of nonhistone protein, thus disturbing chromatin contacts [10]. Histone tail acetylation usually promotes the transcription and is a feature of euchromatin; by contrast, histone tail methylation has usually an inhibitory role for transcription and is a feature of heterochromatin.

The family of ncRNA includes a large set of RNAs like the well-known microRNA (miRNA) or the less known long noncoding RNA (lnRNA) and tRNA fragments (tRF) among others [11]. NcRNAs are involved in the control of gene expression and in the regulation of many biological functions in several tissues;

their expression rate is affected by environmental cues; thus, their expression rate changes in health and disease. Furthermore, the detection of ncRNA in biological fluids makes them a possible epigenetic biomarker for the prognosis, the diagnosis, and the treatment of diseases [12–14].

Thus, an epigenetic machinery comprising various writers, readers, and erasers that have unique structures, functions, and modes of action like the *de novo* and maintenance DNA methyltransferases, histone acetyltransferases, deacetylases, methyltransferases and demethylases, or the ncRNA biosynthetic pathways has been identified in living organisms [13]. However, additional epigenetic mechanisms such as the delivery among tissues of epigenetic marks within extracellular vesicles, exosomes, or microvesicles are starting to emerge, providing evidence of upcoming communication pathways in which the products of specific cell types may affect the expression rate of specific RNAs in target tissues [15–17].

3. Epigenetics in health and disease

In mammals, epigenetic signature is firstly defined in the embryo [18, 19], but this mark is deeply remodeled during the life course as a direct consequence of environmental cues and lifestyle which includes diet, stress, pollutants, smoking, endocrine-disrupting chemicals, physical activity, sedentary life, etc. Therefore, genome activity is epigenetically modulated under exogenous influence, and the environment-dependent changes in gene activity stably propagate from one generation of cells to the next one. Epigenetic changes impact genome functions, thus affecting health and disease status and also behavior; aging-related diseases, cancer, immunity and related disorders, obesity, metabolic disorders, infertility, and cardiovascular and neurological diseases represent only few examples of environmentally dependent diseases, and the literature in the field is growing up day by day [20–35].

Individual health or disease status strongly depends on epigenetic marks, but "parental experiences" may be epigenetically transmitted to the offspring, thus causing trans-generational epigenetic inheritance and affecting offspring health. Such a process requires the transmission of epigenetic marks through gametes and influences fertilization, embryo development, embryo gene expression, and phenotype [36]. Particularly interesting is the possibility that spermatozoa may use ncRNAs as carrier of paternal experiences, thus providing an "epigenetic memory" capable of affecting embryo development and health with consequences on adult offspring phenotype [13, 32, 33].

4. Conclusions and future perspectives

Taken together, both environment and lifestyle deeply affect DNA functions, and their influence may be transmitted to the next generations with consequences on health status. However, experimental data point out that epigenetic marks, and in particular circulating ncRNAs, may represent upcoming biomarkers for the prevention, the diagnosis, and the treatment of diseases, due to the great potential laying in developing epigenetic therapies [37–39].

Author details

Rosaria Meccariello
Dipartimento di Scienze Motorie e del Benessere, Università di Napoli Parthenope, Napoli, Italy

*Address all correspondence to: rosaria.meccariello@uniparthenope.it

IntechOpen

References

[1] Waddington CH. Organizers and Genes. Cambridge: Cambridge Academic; 1940

[2] Waddington CH. Canalization of development and the inheritance of acquired characters. Nature;**150**:563-565

[3] Feinberg AP. Phenotypic plasticity and the epigenetics of human disease. Nature. 2007;**447**:433-440

[4] Kim JK, Samaranayake M, Pradhan S. Epigenetic mechanisms in mammals. Cellular and Molecular Life Sciences. 2009;**66**(4):596-612

[5] Cholewa-Waclaw J, Bird A, von Schimmelmann M, Schaefer A, Yu H, Song H, et al. The role of epigenetic mechanisms in the regulation of gene expression in the nervous system. The Journal of Neuroscience. 2016;**36**(45):11427-11434

[6] Holliday R. DNA methylation and epigenetic mechanisms. Cell Biophysics. 1989;**15**(1-2):15-20

[7] Moore LD, Le T, Fan G. DNA methylation and its basic function. Neuropsychopharmacology. 2013;**38**:23-38

[8] Ferguson-Smith AC. Genomic imprinting: The emergence of an epigenetic paradigm. Nature Reviews. Genetics. 2011;**12**(8):565-575

[9] Bannister AJ, Kouzarides T. Regulation of chromatin by histone modifications. Cell Research. 2011;**21**(3):381-395

[10] Javaid N, Choi N. Acetylation- and methylation-related epigenetic proteins in the context of their targets. Genes (Basel). 2017;**8**(8):196

[11] Palazzo AF, Eliza S, Lee ES. Non-coding RNA: What is functional and what is junk? Frontiers in Genetics. 2015;**6**:2

[12] Taft RJ, Pang KC, Mercer TR, Dinger M, Mattick JS. Non-coding RNAs: Regulators of disease. The Journal of Pathology. 2010;**220**:126-139

[13] Chianese R, Troisi J, Richards S, Scafuro M, Fasano S, Guida M, et al. In reproduction: Epigenetic effects. Current Medicinal Chemistry. 2018;**25**(6):748-770

[14] Kumar P, Kuscu C, Dutta A. Biogenesis and function of transfer RNA-related fragments (tRFs). Trends in Biochemical Sciences. 2016;**41**:679-689

[15] Bakhshandeh B, Kamaleddin MA, Aalishah KA. Comprehensive review on exosomes and microvesicles as epigenetic factors. Current Stem Cell Research & Therapy. 2017;**12**(1):31-36

[16] Qian Z, Shen Q, Yang X, Qiu Y, Zhang W. The role of extracellular vesicles: An epigenetic view of the cancer microenvironment. BioMed Research International. 2015;**2015**:649161

[17] Motti ML, D'Angelo S, Meccariello R. MicroRNAs, cancer and diet: Facts and new exciting perspectives. Current Molecular Pharmacology. 2018;**11**(2):90-96

[18] Seisenberger S, Peat JR, Hore TA, Santos F, Dean W, Reik W. Reprogramming DNA methylation in the mammalian life cycle: Building and breaking epigenetic barriers. Philosophical Transactions of the Royal Society of London. Series B, Biological Sciences. 2013;**368**:20110330

[19] Hogg K, Western PS. Refurbishing the germline epigenome: Out with the old, in with the new. Seminars

in Cell & Developmental Biology. 2015;**45**:104-113

[20] Ling C, Rönn T. Epigeneticsin human obesity and type 2 diabetes. Cell Metabolism. 2019. pii: S1550-4131(19)30137-8

[21] Renani PG, Taheri F, Rostami D, Farahani N, Abdolkarimi H, Abdollahi E, et al. Involvement of aberrant regulation of epigenetic mechanisms in the pathogenesis of Parkinson's disease and epigenetic-based therapies. Journal of Cellular Physiology. 2019. DOI: 10.1002/jcp.28622. [Epub ahead of print]

[22] Rutten MGS, Rots MG, Oosterveer MH. Exploiting epigenetics for the treatment of inborn errors of metabolism. Journal of Inherited Metabolic Disease. 2019. DOI: 10.1002/jimd.12093. [Epub ahead of print]

[23] Kato M, Natarajan R. Epigenetics and epigenomics in diabetic kidney disease and metabolic memory. Nature Reviews. Nephrology. 2019. DOI: 10.1038/s41581-019-0135-6. [Epub ahead of print]

[24] Grova N, Schroeder H, Olivier JL, Turner JD. Epigenetic and neurological impairments associated with early life exposure to persistent organic pollutants. International Journal of Genomics. 2019;**2019**:2085496. DOI: 10.1155/2019/2085496. eCollection 2019

[25] Al-Hasani K, Mathiyalagan P, El-Osta A. Epigenetics, cardiovascular disease, and cellular reprogramming. Journal of Molecular and Cellular Cardiology. 2019;**128**:129-133

[26] Stylianou E. Epigenetics of chronic inflammatory diseases. Journal of Inflammation Research. 2018;**20**(12): 1-14. DOI: 10.2147/JIR.S129027. eCollection 2019

[27] Richard L, Bennett RL, Licht JD. Targeting epigenetics in cancer.

Annual Review of Pharmacology and Toxicology. 2018;**58**:187-207

[28] Flavahan WA, Gaskell E, Bernstein BE. Epigenetic plasticity and the hallmarks of cancer. Science 2017;**357**(6348):pii: eaal2380

[29] Landgrave-Gómez J, Mercado-Gómez O, Guevara-Guzmán R. Epigenetic mechanisms in neurological and neurodegenerative diseases. Frontiers in Cellular Neuroscience. 2015;**9**:58

[30] Sen P, Shah PP, Nativio R, Berger SL. Epigenetic mechanisms and longevity and aging. Cell. 2016;**166**(4):822-839

[31] Das L, Parbin S, Pradhan N, Kausar C, Patra SK. Epigenetics of reproductive infertility. Frontiers in Bioscience (Scholar Edition). 2017;**9**:509-535

[32] Stuppia L, Franzago M, Ballerini P, Gatta V, Antonucci I. Epigenetics and male reproduction: The consequences of paternal lifestyle on fertility, embryo development, and children lifetime health. Clinical Epigenetics. 2015;**7**:120

[33] Jenkins TG, Aston KI, James ER, Carrell DT. Sperm epigenetics in the study of male fertility, offspring health, and potential clinical applications. Systems Biology in Reproductive Medicine. 2017;**63**(2):69-76

[34] Crews D. Epigenetics and its implications for behavioral neuroendocrinology. Frontiers in Neuroendocrinology. 2008;**29**(3):344-357

[35] Roth TL. Epigenetic mechanisms in the development of behavior: Advances, challenges, and future promises of a new field. Development and Psychopathology. 2013;**25**(4 Pt 2):1279-1291

[36] Daxinger L, Whitelaw E. Understanding transgenerational

epigenetic inheritance via the gametes in mammals. Nature Reviews. Genetics. 2012;**13**(3):153-162

[37] Ahuja N, Sharma AR, Baylin SB. Epigenetic therapeutics: A new weapon in the war against cancer. Annual Review of Medicine. 2016;**67**:73-89

[38] Valdespino V, Valdespino PM. Potential of epigenetic therapies in the management of solid tumors. Cancer Management and Research. 2015;**7**:241-251

[39] Mau T, Yung R. Potential of epigenetic therapies in non-cancerous conditions. Frontiers in Genetics. 2014;**5**:438

Chapter 2

Epigenetic Modifications in Plants under Abiotic Stress

Garima Singroha and Pradeep Sharma

Abstract

Plants face a plethora of biotic and abiotic stresses ranging from extreme temperatures to salinity, drought, nutritional deficiencies, chemical toxicity, and pathogen attacks. As a consequence, plants have acquired several sophisticated regulatory mechanisms that allow them to cope with such adverse conditions. Epigenetic regulation plays a key role in the mechanisms of plant response to the environment, without altering DNA sequences. Epigenetics refers to heritable alterations in chromatin architecture that do not involve changes in the underlying DNA sequence but alter gene expression through DNA methylation or histone modifications. The epigenetic regulation of the plant genome is a highly dynamic process that fine-tunes the expression of a pertinent set of genes under certain environmental or developmental conditions. Over the past two decades rapid advancements in the field of high throughput sequencing unveil epigenetic information at genome wide level in various plant species. In view of the adverse effects of global climatic change, utilizing epigenetic differences for developing improved crop varieties is of paramount importance.

Keywords: histone modification, DNA methylation, abiotic stress, chromatin

1. Introduction

Plants being sessile organisms are being constantly challenged by various biotic and abiotic stresses. In order to adapt themselves to the changing environments they need constant changes at molecular level. These efficient and effective controls are provided by epigenetic regulations which improve the survivability of plants by increasing their tolerance toward stress [1, 2]. It is now evident that heritable phenotypic variation does not need to be based on DNA sequence polymorphism [2, 3]. These epigenetic regulations involve different chemical modifications at molecular level that influence gene expression. Epigenetic as defined by Conrad Waddington, is "the study of mitotically and/or meiotically heritable changes in gene function that cannot be explained by changes in DNA sequence" [4]. Today epigenetic refers mainly to the changes that do not relate to the changes in DNA sequence but to chemical modification that can be inherited from one generation to the next [5, 6]. Three types of epigenetic regulatory mechanisms viz. DNA methylation, histone modification and RNA interference (RNAi) are exploited by plants in order to survive adverse conditions.

DNA methylation is a chemical modification, catalyzed by cytosine methyltransferases which involves addition of a methyl group in a DNA sequence onto the cytosine residue in a sequence specific manner, primarily within CpG dinucleotide [7, 8]. The added methyl group provides platform for attachment of various protein complexes that modifies the histone scaffolds resulting in altered gene expression.

In eukaryotic nuclei DNA is organized in the form of nucleosome where it is wrapped around by histone proteins. Histones comprise a family of highly conserved globular proteins whose N-terminal tails are exposed on the surface of the nucleosome octamer for chemical modifications. Histones offer a wealth of post-translational modifications (PTMs) that physically regulate the accessibility of the transcriptional machinery to certain genomic regions, making loci more or less permissive for transcription [9]. Histone modifications include acetylation, methylation, sumoylation, ubiquitination and phosphorylation of histone proteins. Acetylation and phosphorylation are mostly associated with induced gene expression while on the other hand modifications like sumoylation and biotinylation represses gene expression [10, 11]. Such modifications not only impinge on DNA accessibility, but also on the recruitment of specific proteins involved in several processes, including transcription, DNA replication and repair. Histone proteins are not only modified, but can also be replaced by histone variants with different physical properties, or released, in order to allow gene expression [12].

In epigenetic cross-talks diverse classes of noncoding RNA (e.g., small RNAs and long noncoding RNAs) can also modify chromatin structure and silence transcription through formation of RNA scaffolds mediating the recruitment of histone and DNA methyltransferases [13]. RNAi is a sequence specific gene regulation mechanism that acts as a barrier against viruses but also regulates gene expression. In plants RNA interference pathways are mediated by siRNA, miRNA and lncRNA (long non coding RNA). These RNAs are synthesized as 20–30 nucleotide, single stranded molecules from double stranded RNA precursors.

Activation of one or more of these pathways results into changes in chromatin architecture and impacts gene expression. Open chromatin form or closed

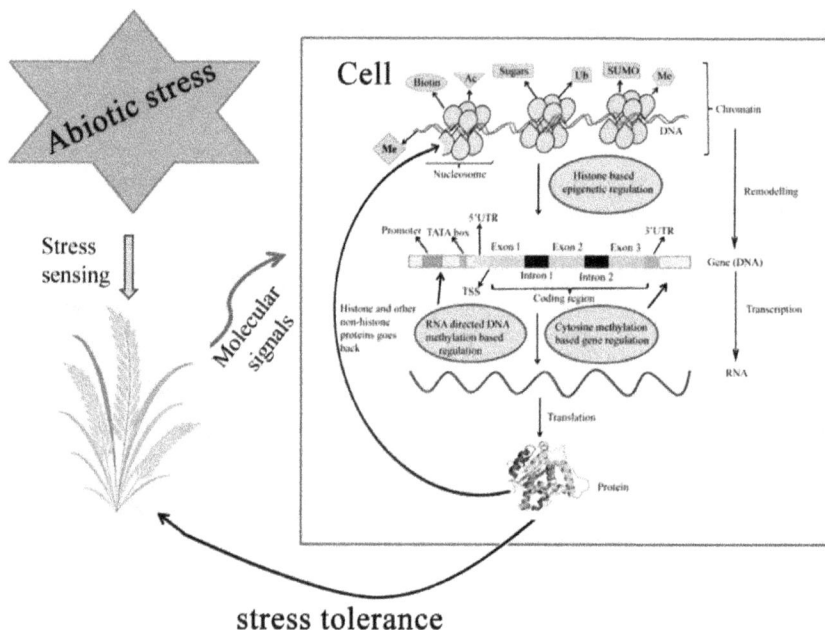

Figure 1.
Various types of epigenetic modifications under stress conditions.

chromatin conformation is associated with gene activation or silencing respectively and governs the onset of gene expression in cells under different developmental or environmental stimuli [14–16]. Transitions from open to close and crosstalk between different epigenetic mechanisms are vital to ensure proper cell function at different developmental stages and under abiotic stress conditions [17–19]. Different types of epigenetic modifications under abiotic stresses have been presented in **Figure 1**.

In the recent years, numerous studies performed toward the characterization of the epigenomic regulation of stress responses in plants have added to our understanding of how diverse abiotic stresses affect chromatin modifications, with their respective transcriptional and physiological implications.

2. Different types of epigenetic modifications

2.1 DNA methylation modification

DNA methylation arises as a result of addition of a methyl group to the nitrogenous base in the DNA strand in a sequence specific manner. DNA methylation occurs at the fifth carbon position of a cytosine ring. Methylation of cytosine leads to the generation of 5-methyl cytosine. On the basis of the target sequence, methylation is classified either as symmetrical or asymmetrical methylation. CG and CHG methylation are termed as symmetrical and CHH methylation as asymmetrical. In plants DNA methylation occurs in all three sequence contexts; the symmetric CG and CHG context and asymmetric CHH (H = A, C or T) context [20]. Plants methylate only some genes and this methylation is usually restricted to CGs located within the gene body while Transposable Element sequences tend to be methylated at most of their CG, CHG, and CHH sites. Methylation in transposable elements and promoter region of a gene leads to silencing on the other hand methylation inside gene body induce gene expression [21]. Thus DNA methylation results into following (i) methylcytosines in the gene body play an important role in regulating the gene expression and (ii) methylcytosines in repetitive sequences (transposable elements), are thought to prevent repetitive sequences from compromising normal genome function [20, 21]. Increased methylation of genomic DNA down regulates gene expression. Down regulated gene expression enable the plants to conserve energy for the sake of biotic or abiotic stress. In contrast, the reduction in methylation of resistance-related genes favors chromatin activation and the expression of novel genes, which provides long-term or permanent resistance for stress.

2.2 Histone modifications in plants

In addition to DNA methylation, histone N-terminal tail modifications constitute an attractive area in epigenetics [22]. Plants contain several histone variants and enzymes that posttranslationally modify histones and influence gene regulation. Application of chromatin immunoprecipitation followed by deep sequencing has given insight into the genome-wide distribution of histone variants and histones bearing different posttranslational modifications [22, 23]. Histone proteins are wrapped around DNA and forms a highly compact structure called nucleosome. Nucleosomes are composed of histone octamers that comprise two copies each of H2A, H2B, H3, and H4. A total of 147 base pair of DNA sequence is wrapped around the histone core. The N termini of histone proteins called N terminal tails undergo various chemical modifications like methylation or acetylation. Such histone modifications are associated with either gene repression or gene activation [24, 25].

In plants methylation and deacetylation of H3K9 and H3K27 results into gene repression whereas acetylation and methylation of H3K4 and H3K36 is associated with gene activation and thus induces gene expression [26]. These covalent modifications in response to various environmental stresses regulates the transcription of wrapped DNA sequence by altering the packaging structure which either activates the DNA for the transcription or makes the structure more condensed so that transcription machinery is unable to reach it.

2.2.1 Histone acetylation/deacetylation

Addition of acetyl group to the N terminal Lysine of histones results into transcriptional activation of a DNA sequence [27]. Acetylation of N terminal lysine causes reduction in the net positive charge of histone and as a result the electrostatic force of attraction between the negatively charged DNA and positively charged histone reduces which leads to the loosening of chromatin and transcriptional activation of DNA [28]. The addition of acetyl group to Lysine is catalyzed by histone acetyltransferases (HATs). Five types of HATs have been identified in eukaryotes viz. GNAT—GCN5-related N-terminal acetyltransferase; MYST—MOZ, Ybf2/Sas3, Sas2, and Tip60; CBP—CREB binding protein; TFII250—TATA binding protein-associated factors and the nuclear hormone-related HATs family. Only specific lysines in a histone protein are acetylated. In different histone proteins different lysine residues undergo modifications for instance, lysine residues of H4 (K5, K8, K12, K16, and K20) and histone H3 (K9, K14, K18, K23, and K27) are subjected to acetylation modifications [29, 30].

2.2.2 Histone methylation

Arginine and Lysine amino acids in histone proteins undergo methylation. Different arginine and lysine residues in different histones undergo different types of methylation (R3 of H2A, R3, K20 of H4 and K4, K9, K27, K36, R2, and R17 of H3 etc.) and these residues can be mono, di or tri methylated. Usually, arginine undergoes mono- and dimethylation only while lysine can undergo mono, di and tri methylation. Methylation can either activate or deactivate a gene depending on the nature of residues methylated for example H3K4 trimethylation activates transcription on the other hand K9 and K27 dimethylation in H3 acts as a repressor [31]. Methylation affects the hydrophobicity of the histone and hence may change histone DNA interactions or may create binding site for various proteins which restricts the binding of transcription machinery and prevents transcription. Histone lysine methyltransferases (HKMT) and protein arginine methyltransferases (PRMT) catalyze methylation of lysine and arginine residues respectively [32].

2.3 miRNA directed DNA methylation

RNA directed DNA methylation (RdDM) is *de novo* cytosine methylation primarily within the region of RNA-DNA sequence identity. Although RdDM pathway can methylate all sequence contexts, but it specifically methylates CHH sequences. The reason for this is that symmetrical methylation is maintained by maintenance methylation each time the DNA is replicated whereas the CHH methylation at many silenced loci is dependent on RNA-guided *de novo* methylation [33].

The 24-nt siRNAs are generated by DNA dependent RNA polymerase Pol IV enzyme, in association with RNA-dependent RNA polymerase 2 (RDR2), and processed by dicer-like 3 (DCL3) [34]. One strand of the resulting 24-nt dsRNA fragments is loaded onto argonaute 4 (AGO4) leading to generation of a silencing effector complex. DNA methylation at sites having sequence homology to the siRNA is dependent on, Pol V, which is a DNA dependent RNA polymerase that transcribes non-coding RNAs. Transcription of Pol V is facilitated by a chromatin remodeling protein which is defective in RNA-directed DNA methylation 1 (DRD1) [35]. KOW domain transcription factor1 (KTF1) which is an adaptor protein, mediates binding of AGO4 and AGO4-bound siRNAs onto the transcripts generated by Pol V forming a silencing effector. This effector acts as signal for DRM2 to introduce methylation at target sites [35]. Development of stress tolerant crop has successfully been achieved by the use of RNAi technology. Transgenic rice plants with tolerance to drought were developed by silencing of activated C-kinase1 receptor [36].

3. Epigenetic changes in crops against abiotic stresses

Due to the unpredictable climate change, crop plants are frequently exposed to a variety of abiotic stresses resulting in reduced crop productivity. Analysis of the stress-associated genes and their regulation in response to the stress can be utilized to enhance understanding of the plant's ability to adapt under changing climatic conditions. DNA methylation and/or histone modifications are influenced by abiotic/biotic factors resulting in the better adaptability of the plants to the adverse environmental conditions. Such epigenetic modifications provide a mechanistic basis for stress memory, which enables plants to respond more effectively and efficiently to the recurring stress as well as to prepare the offspring for potential future assaults.

3.1 Salt-induced epigenetic changes in crop plants

Environmental stresses result in hyper or hypomethylation of DNA. Evidence implicates epigenetic mechanisms in modulating gene expression in plants under abiotic stress. Promoter and gene-body methylation plays important role in regulating gene expression in genotype and organ specific manner under salt stress conditions. Song et al. [37] observed that DNA methylation and histone modifications may have a combined effect on stress inducible gene as salinity stress was reported to affect the expression of various transcription factors in soybean. Ferreira et al., [38] emphasized that hypomethylation in response to salt stress may be correlated with altered expression of DNA demethylases. In another report [39] contrasting differences in cytosine methylation patterns were observed in salinity tolerant wheat cultivar SR3 and its progenitor upon salinity stress imposition. The responses of contrasting wheat genotypes under salt stress could be attributed to the altered expression levels of high affinity potassium transporters (HKTs) regulated through genetic and/or epigenetic mechanisms [40]. It was found that the coding region of high affinity potassium transporters (HKTs) showed variations in 5-mC content in the contrasting wheat genotypes. Salt stress significantly increased methylation level in wheat genotypes. Cytosine residues in CG context were all methylated, whereas increase in 5-mC was observed in CHG and CHH contexts in the shoot of a salt-sensitive wheat genotype under the stress. Variations in chromatin structure (facilitated through histone modifications) also play important role in salt tolerance. Kaldis et al. [41] reported that in *Arabidopsis thaliana* the transcriptional adaptor ADA2b (a modulator of histone acetyltransferases activity) is responsible for its hypersensitivity to salt stress. However, histone modifications are reversible and cross-talk between histone acetylation and cytosine methylation makes the plant responses more complex. Thus, salt stress affects genome-wide DNA methylation as well as histone modifications and these processes are linked to each other for synchronized action against salt stress [42].

3.2 Heat induced epigenetic changes in crop plants

Naydenov, [43] reported that upregulated epigenetic modulators like DRM2, nuclear RNA polymerase D1 (NRPD1) and NRPE1 may be responsible for increased genome methylation in *Arabidopsis thaliana* under heat stress conditions. Heat stress related study in rice showed reduction in seed size which is controlled by OsFIE1 (fertilization independent endosperm). Folsom and coworkers [44] in their study reported that DNA methylation and histone (H3K9me2) methylation are the two major factors governing the expression of OsFIE1. It was found that under heat stress both DNA methylation as well as histone methylation showed a decline (DNA methylation declined by 8.8% and 6.6% with respect to CH and CHG context). Reduced methylation levels resulted into lower expression of OsFIE1 and lead to reduction in rice seed size. Histone modifications like acetylation have also been reported to occur under heat stress conditions. At high temperatures, a histone variant H2A.Z causes transcriptional changes in stress responsive genes [45]. Mutations in a gene *GCN5* that codes for histone acetyltransferase, resulted in impaired transcriptional activation of heat stress responsive genes like HSAF3 and MBF1c and lead to thermal susceptibility of *Arabidopsis thaliana* [46]. The duration of heat treatment also has diverse effects on the epigenetic mechanisms emphasizing complexity in the epigenetic regulation of heat stress [47].

3.3 Epigenetic modifications in response to drought

Drought stress conditions generally tend to increase demethylation. It is also observed that DNA methylation shows tissue specificity. In *Oryza sativa* drought induced a total of 12.1% methylation differences accounted across different tissues, genotype and developmental stages. The overall DNA methylation level at the same developmental stage was lesser in roots than in leaves indicating significant role of roots under water insufficiency [48]. Correlation between DNA methylation and drought stress tolerance has been shown in lowland and drought-tolerant rice cultivars. IR20, a drought susceptible variety, undergoes hypomethylation under drought conditions whereas the tolerant varieties "PMK3" and "Paiyur" showed hypermethylation. These changes in methylation pattern contributed to differential expression of stress responsive genes [49]. In another study conducted in rice it was illustrated that hypomethylation has significant role in the drought tolerant attribute of rice genotypes [50].

In several studies the abundance in transcript levels of drought responsive gene was correlated with changes in histone modification. Under drought conditions several histone alterations like acetylation, methylation, phosphorylation and sumoylation occurs [51]. Reports have documented that drought stress response is memorized through histone modification of various drought stress induced genes [52]. In a study in *A. thaliana* it was shown that an increase in H3K4 trimethylation and H3K9 acetylation on the promoter region and H3K23 and H3K27 acetylation on the coding regions is responsible for drought-induced expression of stress-responsive genes [53]. Under stress conditions, accumulation of transcripts of stress responsive genes was positively correlated with histone modifications H3K9ac and H3K4me3 as both are marks of an active state of gene expression [54].

3.4 Epigenetic modifications in response to cold

Upon imposition of cold stress HDACs are upregulated that results into deacetylation of H3 and H4 and successively heterochromatic tandem repeats get activated [55, 56]. This results into reduction of DNA methylation and histone (H3K9me2) methylation at the targeted region of maize genome [39, 57]. In a study conducted on the effect of cold on maize seedlings it was found that cold stress induced genome wide DNA methylation in root tissues except only in a 1.8-kb segment designated as ZmMI1. Under normal conditions ZmMI1 segment is methylated but under chilling conditions it is demethylated. This segment is representative of a stress responsive gene that plays role under stress conditions [58].

Even after 7 days of recovery, cold induced hypomethylation was not reverted back. In a similar study conducted by Saraswat et al. of DNA methylation pattern in cold grown maize 28 differentially amplified fragments were obtained. *In silico* analysis of these fragments revealed their role in several processes like photosynthesis, hormone regulation and in cold response [59]. A recent study in apple highlighted the importance of epigenetic changes in response to dormancy caused by low temperature. High chilling conditions decreased total methylation that lead to reinitiation of active growth and subsequent fruit set in apple [60, 61].

4. Techniques for deciphering epigenetic changes in plants

4.1 Histone modifications

4.1.1 Chromatin immunoprecipitation (ChiP) techniques

This technique is used to assay DNA–protein binding under *in vivo* conditions. This involves shearing genomic DNA into smaller fragments through sonication to generate fragments ranging 200–800 base pairs. Gentle formaldehyde treatment is given to crosslink proteins with DNA. Antibodies raised specifically for protein of interest are used to precipitate the protein-DNA complex. Precipitated DNA thus obtained is released by acid treatment and amplified by PCR [62].

4.1.2 ChiP-Seq

Advancements in the field of next-generation sequencing have made it possible to combines ChiP with next-generation sequencing technology such as Solexa. ChiP-Seq combines Chromatin immunoprecipitation and sequencing technologies to decipher genome wide distribution of histone proteins [62].

4.1.3 ChiP PCR

Immunoprecipitated DNA is amplified and quantified by real time PCR (RT-PCR) using TaqMan or Syber Green Technologies with specified primers for analysis of specific genomic regions associated with particular histones.

4.2 DNA methylation profiling in plants

Earlier studies focused on determining methylation status of the gene of interest. With the use of microarray hybridization technology DNA methylation has been scaled up to genome wide level. Next generation sequencing platforms are now being used for the construction of genomic maps of DNA methylation at single-base resolution.

4.2.1 Genome-wide bisulfite sequencing

Bisulfite treatment converts unmethylated cytosines to uracil, allowing for the identification of methylated cytosines by comparing a treated sample to a reference sample [63]. Bisulfite sequencing evaluates individual cytosines in a target sequence for essentially all cytosines in a genome (i.e. whole-genome bisulfate sequencing or WGBS).

4.2.2 Methylated DNA immunoprecipitation (MeDIP)

Genomic DNA is fragmented and precipitated with 5-methylcytosine-specific antibody. The precipitated DNA is then analyzed by PCR or whole genome tiling microarrays [64, 65].

4.2.3 Reduced-representation bisulfite sequencing (RRBS)

RRBS came into existence for the purpose of deciphering the mammalian methylome at low cost [66]. Bisulfite sequencing can be used for genomic fragments that are isolated with restriction enzymes thus providing single-nucleotide resolution of DNA methylation within each of the fragments. Availability of both sequence and methylation variation from same set of locus allows comparison of genetic and epigenetic differences. It is based on MspI restriction digestion and selection of (40 and 220 basepair) digested fragments for bisulfite conversion and sequencing [67]. RRBS has been adopted for plant population studies and can be applied to species for which no reference genomes are available [68, 69]. RRBS has also been used in oak populations [70] and *Brassica rapa* [71].

4.2.4 Shotgun bisulfite sequencing

This combines bisulfite treatment of genomic DNA with next generation sequencing technology such as Solexa sequencing. The converted sequences are mapped to the reference genome sequence to identify methyl-cytosines [63, 72].

5. Conclusions

In view of the increasing stress conditions experienced by plants due to global climatic changes, epigenetics is considered as an important regulatory mechanism that is influenced by environmental stimulus. This regulatory mechanism is of utmost significant importance in terms of its inheritance over generations. Advancements in the ultra-high-throughput techniques have revolutionized identification of epigenetic changes and improved our knowledge on effect of epigenetic changes on regulation of gene expression. Manipulation of DNA (de) methylation level at specific loci may allow us to regulate gene expression and the neighboring chromatin states, impacting cell physiology and biochemistry. Therefore, one of the possible, yet unexplored, ways to improve stress tolerance in crop plants may be to augment stress memory of the plants by targeted modification of the epigenome. Thus utilizing epigenetic variation for developing improved abiotic stress tolerant crop verities is an undertaking of paramount importance.

Acknowledgements

Authors would like to thank Director ICAR-Indian Institute of Wheat and Barley Research.

Conflict of interest

The authors hereby declare that there is no conflict of interest.

Abbreviations

DNA	deoxyribonucleic acid
RNAi	ribonucleic acid interference
PTMs	post-transcriptional modifications
H3K9	histone 3, 9th lysine
H3K27	histone 3, 27th lysine
HATs	histone acetyltransferases
HKMT	histone lysine methyl transferases
PRMT	protein arginine methyl transferases
nt	nucleotide
RDR2	RNA-dependent RNA polymerase 2
siRNAs	small interfering ribonucleic acid
AGO4	argonaute 4
dsRNA	double stranded ribonucleic acid
HKTs	high affinity potassium transporters
NRPD1	nuclear RNA polymerase D1
OsFIE1	fertilization independent endosperm
PCR	polymerase chain reactions
WGBS	whole-genome bisulfate sequencing
MeDIP	methylated DNA immunoprecipitation
RRBS	reduced representation bisulfite sequencing

Author details

Garima Singroha* and Pradeep Sharma
ICAR-Indian Institute of Wheat and Barley Research (IIWBR),
Karnal, Haryana, India

*Address all correspondence to: garima.singroha@gmail.com

IntechOpen

References

[1] Hirayama T, Shinozaki K. Research on plant abiotic stress responses in the post-genome era: Past, present and future. Plant Journal. 2010;**61**(6):1041-1052

[2] Richards EJ. Inherited epigenetic variation–Revisiting soft inheritance. Nature Reviews Genetics. 2006;7:395-401

[3] Bossdorf O, Richards CL, Pigliucci M. Epigenetics for ecologists. Ecology Letters. 2008;**11**:106-115

[4] Waddington CH. The epigenotype. Endeavour. 1942;**1**:18-20

[5] Fujimoto R, Sasaki T, Ishikawa R, Osabe K, Kawanabe T, Dennis ES. Molecular mechanisms of epigenetic variation in plants. International Journal of Molecular Sciences. 2012;**13**(8):9900-9922

[6] Feng S, Jacobsen SE, Reik W. Epigenetic reprogramming in plant and animal development. Science. 2010;**330**:622-627

[7] Niederhuth CE, Schmitz RJ. Putting DNA methylation in context: From genomes to gene expression in plants. Biochimica et Biophysica Acta. 2017;**1860**:149-156

[8] Bewick AJ, Ji L, Niederhuth CE, Willing EM, Hofmeister BT, Shi X, et al. On the origin and evolutionary consequences of gene body DNA methylation. Proceedings of the National Academy of Sciences of the United States of America. 2016;**113**:9111

[9] Kouzarides T. Chromatin modifications and their function. Cell. 2007;**23, 128**(4):693-705

[10] Nathan D, Ingvarsdottir K, Sterner DE, Bylebyl GR, Dokmanovic M, Dorsey JA, et al. Histone sumoylation is a negative regulator in *Saccharomyces cerevisiae* and shows dynamic interplay with positive-acting histone modifications. Genes & Development. 2006;**20**:966-976

[11] Camporeale G, Oommen AM, Griffin JB, Sarath G, Zempleni J. K12-biotinylated histone H4 marks heterochromatin in human lymphoblastoma cells. The Journal of Nutritional Biochemistry. 2007;**18**:760-768

[12] Johnson LM, Cao X, Jacobsen SE. Interplay between two epigenetic marks: DNA methylation and histone H3 lysine 9 methylation life science core curriculum 2 molecular, cell and developmental. Current Biology. 2002;**12**:1360-1367. DOI: 10.1016/S0960-9822(02)00976-4

[13] Holoch D, Moazed D. RNA-mediated epigenetic regulation of gene expression. Nature. 2015;**16**:71-84

[14] Berger SL. The complex language of chromatin regulation duringtranscription. Nature. 2007;**447**(7143):407-412

[15] Forderer A, Zhou Y, Turck p F. The age of multiplexicity: Recruitement and interactions of polycomb complexes in plants. Current opinions in Plant Biology. 2016;**29**:169-178

[16] Du J, Johnson LM, Jacobsen SE, Patel DJ. DNA methylation pathways and their crosstalk with histone methylation. Nature Reviews Molecular Cell Biology. 2015;**16**(9):519-532

[17] Chen Z, Zhang H, Jablonowski D, Zhou X, Ren X, Hong X, et al. Mutations in ABO1/ELO2, a subunit of holo-elongator, increase abscisic acid sensitivity and drought tolerance in *Arabidopsis thaliana*. Molecular and Cellular Biology. 2006;**26**:6902-6912

[18] Li X, Zhu J, Hu F, Ge S, Ye M, Xiang H, et al. Singlebase resolution maps of cultivated and wild rice methylomes and regulatory roles of DNA methylation in plant gene expression. BMC Genomics. 2012;**13**:300

[19] Lu X, Wang W, Ren W, Chai Z, Guo W. Genome-wide epigenetic regulation of gene transcription in maize seeds. PLoS One. 2015;**10**:1-20. DOI: 10.1371/journal.pone.0139582

[20] Miura A, Yonebayashi S, Watanabe K, Toyama T, Shimada H, Kakutani T. Mobilization of transposons by a mutation abolishing full DNA methylation in *Arabidopsis*. Nature. 2001;**411**:212-214

[21] Simon W, Henderson I, Jacobsen S. Gardening the genome: DNA methylation in *Arabidopsis thaliana*. Nature Reviews Genetics. 2005;**6**:351-360

[22] Berger SL, Kouzarides T, Shiekhattar R, Shilatifard A. An operational definition of epigenetics. Genes & Development. 2009;**23**:781-783

[23] Roudier F, Teixeira FK, Colot V. Chromatin indexing in Arabidopsis: An epigenomic tale of tails and more. Trends in Genetics. 2009;**25**:511-517

[24] Roudier F, Ahmed I, Berard C, Sarazin A, Mary-Huard T, Cortijo S, et al. Integrative epigenomic mapping defines four main chromatin states in Arabidopsis. The EMBO Journal. 2011;**30**:1928-1938

[25] He G, Elling AA, Deng XW. The epigenome and plant development. Annual Review of Plant Biology. 2011;**62**:411-435

[26] Lauria M, Rossi V. Epigenetic control of gene regulation in plants. Biochimica et Biophysica Acta. 2011;**1809**:369-378

[27] Fuchs J, Demidov D, Houben A, Schubert I. Chromosomal histone modification patterns–From conservation to diversity. Trends in Plant Science. 2006;**11**:199-208

[28] Shahbazian MD, Grunstein M. Functions of site-specific histone acetylation and deacetylation. Annual Review of Biochemistry. 2007;**76**:75-100

[29] Sterner DE, Berger SL. Acetylation of histones and transcription-related factors. Microbiology and Molecular Biology Reviews. 2000;**64**:435-459

[30] Earley KW, Shook MS, Brower-Toland B, Hicks L, Pikaard CS. In vitro specificities of *Arabidopsis* co-activator histone acetyltransferases: Implications for histone hyperacetylation in gene activation. The Plant Journal. 2007;**52**:615-626

[31] Tamaru H, Selker EU. A histone H3 methyltransferase controls DNA methylation in *Neurospora crassa*. Nature. 2001;**414**(6861):277-283

[32] Kanno T, Bucher E, Daxinger L, Huettel B, Kreil DP, Breinig F, et al. RNA-directed DNA methylation and plant development require an IWR1-type transcription factor. EMBO Reports. 2010;**11**:65-71

[33] Matzke M, Kanno T, Daxinger L, Huettel B, Matzke AJ. RNA-mediated chromatin-based silencing in plants. Current Opinion in Cell Biology. 2009;**21**:367-376

[34] He XJ, Hsu YF, Zhu S, Wierzbicki AT, Pontes O, Pikaard CS, et al. An effector of RNA directed DNA methylation in *Arabidopsis* is an ARGONAUTE 4-and RNA-binding protein. Cell. 2009;**137**(3):498-508

[35] Naumann U, Daxinger L, Kanno T, Eun C, Long Q, Lork-ovic ZJ, et al. Genetic evidence that DNA methyltransferase DRM2 has a direct catalytic role in RNA directed DNA

methylation in *Arabidopsis thaliana*. Genetics. 2011;**187**(3):977-979

[36] Tang N, Ma S, Zong W, Yang N, Lv Y, Yan C, et al. MODD mediates deactivation and degradation of OsbZIP46 to negatively regulate ABA signaling and drought resistance in rice. The Plant Cell. 2016;**28**:2161-2177

[37] Song Y, Ji D, Li S, Wang P, Li Q, Xiang F. The dynamic changes of DNA methylation and histone modifications of salt responsive transcription factor genes in soybean. PLoS One. 2012;**7**(7):e41274

[38] Ferreira LJ, Azevedo V, Maroco J, Oliveira MM, Santos AP. Salt tolerant and sensitive rice varieties display differential methylome flexibility under salt stress. PLoS One. 2015;**10**(5):e0124060

[39] Wang W, Zhao X, Pan Y, Zhu L, Fu B, Li Z. DNA methylation changes detected by methylation-sensitive amplified polymorphism in two contrasting rice genotypes under salt stress. Journal of Genetics and Genomics. 2011;**38**(9):419-424

[40] Kumar S, Beena AS, Awana M, Singh A. Salt-induced tissue-specific cytosine methylation downregulates expression of HKT genes in contrasting wheat (*Triticum aestivum L.*) genotypes. DNA and Cell Biology. 2017;**36**:283-394

[41] Kaldis A, Tsementzi D, Tanriverdi O, Vlachonasios KE. *Arabidopsis thaliana* transcriptional co-activators ADA2 band SGF29a are implicated in salt stress responses. Planta. 2011;**233**:749-762

[42] Pandey G, Sharma N, Sahu PP, Prasad M. Chromatin-based epigenetic regulation of plant abiotic stress response. Current Genomics. 2016;**17**:490-498

[43] Naydenov M, Baev V, Apostolova E, Gospodinova N, Sablok G, Gozmanova M, et al. High-temperature effect on genes engaged in DNA methylation and affected by DNAmethylation in *Arabidopsis*. Plant Physiology and Biochemistry. 2015;**87**:102-108

[44] Folsom JJ, Begcy K, Hao X, Wang D, Walia H. Rice fertilization-independent endosperm1 regulates seed size under heat stress by controlling early endosperm development. Plant Physiology. 2014;**165**(1):238-248

[45] Kim JM, Sasaki T, Sako K, Seki M. Chromatin changes in response to drought, salinity, heat, and cold stresses in plants. Frontiers in Plant Science. 2015;**6**:114-119

[46] Hu Z, Song N, Zheng M, Liu X, Liu Z, Xing J, et al. Histone acetyl-transferase GCN5 is essential for heat stress-responsive gene activation and thermo-tolerance in Arabidopsis. The Plant Journal. 2015;**84**(6):1178-1191. DOI: 10.1111/tpj.13076

[47] Liu J, Feng L, Li J, He Z. Genetic and epigenetic control of plant heat responses. Frontiers in Plant Scienecs. 2015;**6**:267

[48] Suji KK, John A. An epigenetic change in rice cultivars underwater stress conditions. Electronic Journal of Plant Breeding. 2010;**1**:1142-1143

[49] Gayacharan AJ. Epigenetic responses to drought stress in rice (*Oryza sativa L.*). Physiology and Molecular Biology of Plants. 2013;**19**(3):379-387

[50] Li D-h, Li H, et al. Down-regulated expression of RACK1 gene by RNA interference enhances drought tolerance in rice. Rice Science. 2009;**16**(1):14-20. DOI: 10.1016/S1672-6308(08)60051-7

[51] Kim JM, To TK, Ishida J, Morosawa T, Kawashima M, Matsui A, et al. Alterations of lysine modifications on the histone H3N-tail under drought stress conditions in *Arabidopsis*

thaliana. Plant & Cell Physiology. 2008;**49**:1580-1588

[52] Chen H-M, Chen L-T, Patel K, Li Y-H, Baulcombe DC, Wu S-H. 22-nucleotide RNAs trigger secondary siRNA biogenesis in plants. Proceedings of the National Academy of Sciences. 2010;**107**:15269-15274

[53] Kim JM, To TK, Ishida J, Matsui A, Kimura H, Seki M. Transition of chromatin status during the process of recovery from drought stress in *Arabidopsis thaliana*. Plant & Cell Physiology. 2012;**53**(5):847-856

[54] van Dijk K, Ding Y, Malkaram S, Riethoven JJ, Liu R, Yang J, et al. Dynamic changes in genome-wide histone H3lysine 4 methylation patterns in response to dehydration stress in Arabidopsis thaliana. BMC Plant Biology. 2010;**10**:238

[55] Ding B, Bellizzi MR, Ning Y, Meyers BC, Wang GL. HDT701, a histone H4 deacetylase, negatively regulates plant innate immunity by modulating histone H4 acetylation of defence related genes in rice. The Plant Cell. 2012;**24**(9):3783-3794

[56] Zhu J, Jeong J, Zhu Y, Sokolchik I, Miyazaki S, Zhu JK, et al. Involvement of *Arabidopsis* HOS15 in histone deacetylation and cold tolerance. Proceedings of the National Academy of Sciences of the United States of America. 2007;**105**:4945-4950

[57] Hu Y, Zhang L, He S, Huang M, Tan J, Zhao L, et al. Cold stress selectively unsilences tandem repeats in heterochromatin associated with accumulation of H3K9ac. Plant, Cell & Environment. 2012;**35**:2130-2142

[58] Hu Y, Zhang L, Zhao L, Li J, He S, Zhou K, et al. Trichostatin a selectively suppresses the cold-induced transcription of the ZmDREB1 gene in maize. PLoS One. 2011;**6**(7):e22132

[59] Steward N, Ito M, Yamaguchi Y, Koizumi N, Sano H. Periodic DNA methylation in maize nucleosomes and demethylation by environmental stress. The Journal of Biological Chemistry. 2002;**277**(40):37741-37746

[60] Saraswat S, Yadav AK, Sirohi P, Singh NK. Role of epigenetics in crop improvement: water and heat stress. Journal of Plant Biology. 2017;**60**:231-240. DOI: 10.1007/s12374-017-0053-8

[61] Kumar G, Rattan UK, Singh A. Chilling mediated DNA methylation changes during dormancy and its release reveal the importance of epigenetic regulation during winter dormancy in apple. PLoS One. 2016;**11**(2):e0149934

[62] Park P. ChIP-seq: Advantages and challenges of a maturing technology. Nature Reviews. Genetics. 2009;**10**:669-680

[63] Cokus SJ, Feng S, Zhang X, Chen Z, Merriman B, Haudenschild CD, et al. Shotgun bisulphite sequencing of the *Arabidopsis* genome reveals DNA methylation patterning. Nature. 2008;**452**:215-219

[64] Zhang X, Yazaki J, Sundaresan A, Cokus S, Chan SW, Chen H, et al. Genomewide high-resolution mapping and functional analysis of DNA methylation in *Arabidopsis*. Cell. 2006;**126**:1189-1201

[65] Zilberman D, Gehring M, Tran RK, Ballinger T, Henikoff S. Genome-wide analysis of *Arabidopsis thaliana* DNA methylation uncovers an interdependence between methylation and transcription. Nature Genetics. 2007;**39**:61-69

[66] Meissner A. Epigenetic modifications in pluripotent and differentiated cells. Nature Biotechnology. 2010;**28**:1079-1088

[67] Gu H, Smith ZD, Bock C, Boyle P, Gnirke A, Meissner A. Preparation

of reduced representation bisulfite sequencing libraries for genome-scale DNA methylation profiling. Nature Protocols. 2011;**6**(4):468-481

[68] Trucchi E, Mazzarella AB, Gilfillan GD, Romero MT, Paun O. BsRADseq screening DNA methylation in natural populations of non-model species. Molecular Ecology. 2016;**25**:1697-1713

[69] van Gurp TP, Wagemaker NCAM, Wouters B, Vergeer P, Ouborg JNJ, Verhoeven KJF. epiGBS: Reference-free reduced representation bisulfite sequencing. Nature Methods. 2016;**13**:322-324

[70] Platt A, Gugger PF, Pellegrini M, Sork VL. Genome-wide signature of local adaptation linked to variable CpG methylation in oak populations. Molecular Ecology. 2015;**24**:3823-3830. DOI: 10.1111/mec.13230

[71] Chen X, Ge X, Wang J, Tan C, King GJ, Liu K. Genome wide DNA methylation profiling modified reduced representation bisulphate sequencing in *Brassica rapa* suggests that epigenetic modifications play a key role in polyploidy genome evaluation. Frontiers in Plant Sciences. 2015;**6**:836

[72] Lister R, O'Malley RC, Tonti-Filippini J, Gregory BD, Berry CC, Millar AH, et al. Highly integrated single-base resolution maps of the epigenome in *Arabidopsis*. Cell. 2008;**133**:523-536

Chapter 3

A Landscape of Epigenetic Regulation by MicroRNAs to the Hallmarks of Cancer and Cachexia: Implications of Physical Activity to Tumor Regression

Gabriel Cardial Tobias, João Lucas Penteado Gomes,
Ursula Paula Renó Soci, Tiago Fernandes
and Edilamar Menezes de Oliveira

Abstract

In the last decades, there has been a remarkable advance in the treatment of most types of cancer, improving the patient's prognosis. During cancer progression, tumor cells develop several biological changes to support initiation, proliferation, and resistance to death. Nearly 50–80% of all oncologic patients experience rapid weight loss that is related to ~20% of cancer-related deaths. Cancer cachexia is a syndrome characterized by loss of skeletal muscle mass, anorexia, and anemia. A lot of effort in scientific investigation has contributed to the understanding of cancer processes, in which epigenetic changes, as microRNAs, can influence cancer progression. Therefore, useful strategies to control the cancer-induced epigenetic changes in the tumor cells can have a key role in a clinical perspective to decrease the cancer development and aggressiveness. Physical activity has been proposed as a suitable tool to manage tumor growth and cachexia and to improve the deleterious sequelae experienced during cancer treatment. Although the molecular mechanisms involved in these responses are poorly understood, this chapter aims to discuss the role of microRNAs in the cancer-induced epigenetic changes and how physical activity could influence the epigenetic control of tumor cells and cachexia and their potential role in clinical applications for cancer.

Keywords: epigenetic, cancer, hallmarks of cancer, cachexia, physical activity, tumor progression, microRNAs

1. Introduction: hallmarks of cancer, genetics and epigenetics

In the last decades, there has been a remarkable advance in the treatment of most types of cancer, improving the patient's prognosis [1]. However, cancer remains the second major cause of death in the world and major cause of death in the rich countries [2, 3]. Cancer consists in a set of diseases characterized by the progressive accumulation of mutations in the cell. These mutations provide changes in the intracellular environment that induce advantages for its proliferation as well as greater resistance to mechanisms of cell death. A dysfunctional cluster of these cells is classically known as tumor. Currently, cancer is understood as a microenvironment, in which the interactions between the cellular elements that compose it are determinants for the progression of the disease. For example, such elements would be involved in the interaction of tumor cells with normal cells such as fibroblasts, adipocytes, immune system cells, and endothelial cells [4–6]. All these cellular interactions support the development of cancer cachexia, which affects approximately 50–80% of cancer patients, and more than 25% of cancer deaths are a direct consequence of cachexia [7]. Cancer cachexia is directly related to a reduction in tolerance to physical effort [8], a reduction in tolerance to cancer treatments [9], and a shorter patient survival [10].

During cancer progression, tumor cells develop a number of important biological changes to support initiation, proliferation, and resistance to death known as cancer hallmarks [5, 6]. Hanahan and Weinberg [5, 6] discuss 10 biological capabilities acquired by tumor cells that may be common among the different neoplasms and are important for the development and growth of the tumor mass, namely: (1) sustaining proliferative signaling, (2) loss of growth suppressors, (3) resisting cell death, (4) enabling replicative immortality, (5) inducing angiogenesis, (6) activating invasion and metastasis, (7) genome instability, (8) inflammation, (9) reprogramming of energy metabolism, and (10) loss of immune destruction [5, 6]. Among the 10 cancer-related biological processes, we point out that 6 are of fundamental importance for tumor mass growth.

1. Sustaining proliferative signaling

    In normal tissues, there is a careful control of the release of growth and proliferation factors for the regulation of the cell cycle, which ensures adequate tissue architecture and function. However, tumor cells show abnormal proliferation signaling, which promote exacerbated cell proliferation that generates morphological and functional tissue disarrangement. Some mutations are shown as probable causes of a normal cell to initiate a sustained proliferation and tumorigenesis. For example, mutation of *PIK3CA* gene and tyrosine kinases are mutations well described that promote sustained proliferation of a tumor cell [11].

2. Loss of growth suppressors.

    Tumor cells bypass growth suppressor signals through the escape of mechanisms that negatively control cell proliferation. Usually, tumor cells show loss of *p53*, a well-known tumor suppressor that controls proliferation, senescence, and cellular apoptotic programs, culminating in the uncontrolled growth of tumor cells. Tumor cells must also bypass powerful programs that negatively regulate cell proliferation; many of these programs depend on the actions of tumor suppressor genes [12].

3. Resisting cell death.

    Over the past few decades, the literature has shown that apoptosis-programmed cell death serves as a natural barrier to the development of cancer. Apoptosis is triggered in response to various physiological stresses that tumor cells undergo during the course of tumorigenesis or as a result of antineoplastic therapies. However, tumor cells have the ability to resist apoptosis and subsequently progress to conditions of malignancy and resistance to therapy [5].

4. Enabling replicative immortality.

    In healthy tissues, most normal cells have growth and cell division capacity controlled, but tumor cells have unlimited replicative potential, which favors the development of tumors [5].

5. Inducing angiogenesis.

    In any tissue, the presence of vessels allows both the uptake of nutrients and oxygen and the release of substances not useful for the cells. Moreover, angiogenesis occurs temporarily in response to some stimulation such as healing and the female reproductive cycle, being a transient process. However, this process is sustained and dysfunctional, since new vessels that present less coverage of pericytes appear continuously, favoring tumor growth [5].

6. Activating invasion and metastasis.

    Tissue invasion and metastasis are probably the most relevant features developed by tumor cells, since the major cause of cancer death is associated with the formation of metastatic tumors. Metastasis is the formation of a new tumor, originating from the primary tumor. This is a complex process in which primary tumor cells invade blood and lymphatic circulation, spreading and forming colonies at distant sites from the primary tumor [13].

To reach the circulation and invade distant tissues, tumor cells need to modify their configuration and undergo a process named epithelial-mesenchymal transition (EMT). Thus, tumor cells with epithelial characteristics deactivate the mechanisms of cell adhesion and acquire locomotor properties, becoming able to infiltrate the stroma and have access to blood and lymphatic vessels [14, 15]. Moreover, for the colonization of tumor cells in distant tissues, the preparation of the *"premetastatic niche,"* which corresponds to the preparation of the metastatic tissue target of the tumor cells, is fundamental. The process of formation of the *premetastatic niche* involves an intricate cellular signaling at the systemic and local level, involving tumor-secreted factors and tumor-shed extracellular vesicle interaction [16]. Additionally, although Hanahan and Weinberg [5, 6] demonstrate possible treatments against hallmarks of cancer, the individual response to various treatments is still unpredictable [17, 18], demonstrating the plasticity of tumor cells [19–23]. The understanding of *premetastatic niche* is a new paradigm for the initiation of metastasis that can enable the clinical body to fight metastasis, and would benefit greatly from understanding the pathological processes occurring before the development of macrometastases [24].

2. Epigenetics and cancer

    Cancer is considered a typically genetic disease; however, epigenetic modifications play an important role in the development and progression of cancer [5, 6, 25–27].

    The term "epigenetics" was originally described by Conrad Waddington to describe hereditary changes in a cell phenotype that were independent of changes in DNA sequence [28].

    Epigenetic modifications reflect a complexity of factors that determine the condensation state of chromatin, which determines whether the DNA is accessible to proteins that control gene transcription. A relaxed or "open" chromatin state allows gene transcription, while a condensed or "closed" chromatin condition prevents gene transcription [25, 26, 28–31]. Epigenetic mechanisms currently believed to play a role in the development of cancer include: (1) DNA methylation of cytosine bases in CG-rich sequences, called CpG islands; (2) posttranslational modification of histones (proteins that form the nucleosomes), which regulate the packaging structure of DNA (called chromatin); and (3) microRNAs (miRs) and noncoding RNAs [25, 26, 28–31].

Although DNA methylation and histone modifications are important components of epigenetic regulation [25, 26, 28–31], here we will focus on the role of alterations in miRs expression, since their expression is regulated through various mechanisms, including epigenetic modifications, and because their functions are aberrant in cancer, boosting the progression of the disease.

3. MicroRNAs

MiRs are a class of molecules that have an important role in the regulation of protein expression, even after the transcription of messenger RNA (mRNA).

MiRs are characterized as small RNAs of approximately 17–22 nucleotides, noncoding proteins, that act by binding to the mRNA, repressing the translation of proteins. MiRs are found in several organisms as animals and plants and control a lot of physiological and pathological processes. Evidence shows that at least one-third of all biological processes are controlled by miRs [32].

This class of molecules was first observed in 1993 by Lee et al., which demonstrated that miR *lin-4* was associated with larval development of *C elegans* [33]. Although the discovery of the first miR occurred in 1993, miRs researches only progressed in the year 2000, when miR *lin-4* was found to participate in the posttranscriptional control of *lin-14* protein through the complementary binding of miR with the 3' untranslated region (3'UTR region) of the protein mRNA [34]. After the pioneering study by Hong et al., many studies have been developed to demonstrate that small RNAs could participate in posttranscriptional controls. Thus, Ambros observed that miR *let-7* had a partially complementary binding to the 3'UTR region of the *lin-4* protein mRNA, negatively controlling its protein expression [34, 35]. These findings led to the discovery of new miRs, and more than 30,000 mature miRs are now known in the most diverse organisms [32].

As mentioned, miRs exert their action through partially or totally binding to the 3'UTR region of the target mRNA. The complete complementarity induces the degradation of the mRNAs, being commonly observed in plants. In mammals, there is partial complementarity, which inhibits the translation of the target transcript [36].

The miRs bind their *seed* region, that in mammals comprises 2–8 nucleotide, with the target mRNA, present in the 3'UTR region, where only some of the base pairs are complementary. Due to the imperfect pairing and small size of these molecules, there is the possibility of an miR presenting various targets [36].

The biogenesis of miRs begins with the action of the enzyme RNA polymerase II that generates a primary transcript called pri-miR. The pri-miR has a hairpin double helix structure with approximately 300 nucleotides. Still in the cell nucleus, the Drosha enzyme and its cofactor DGCR8 cleave the pri-miR, forming its precursor, the pre-miR. The pre-miR is exported to the cytosol by the exportin 5 enzyme. In the cytoplasm, the pre-miR is cleaved by the enzyme dicer, originating two strands together, one being the mature miR and the other called an antisense. Dicer cleaves again and separates the duplex. The mature miR is then incorporated by a multimeric complex named RISC that contains argonaute protein (AGO) as showed in **Figure 1**, while the other strand can be degraded or incorporated in other RISC complex to exert negative regulation of target mRNAs [32].

Recently, the interest in the study of miRs has increased, since they exert a paracrine function and are effective in the tissue communication. Also, an miR can exert the same function on different cell types, as different function in the same cells. In 2008, the presence of miRs in plasma and other biological fluids was discovered, demonstrating that miRs are viable in the extracellular environment and important signaling molecules. There are circulating miRs in almost all biological fluids, including: milk, plasma, serum, saliva, urine, tear, and amniotic fluid [37]. Circulating miRs are remarkably stable, resistant to RNase activity, freeze-thaw cycles as well as extreme pH. This stability is associated with the carriers that carry them and can be secreted by the cells through different vesicles such as exosomes, HDL, or AGO proteins containing apoptotic bodies [37].

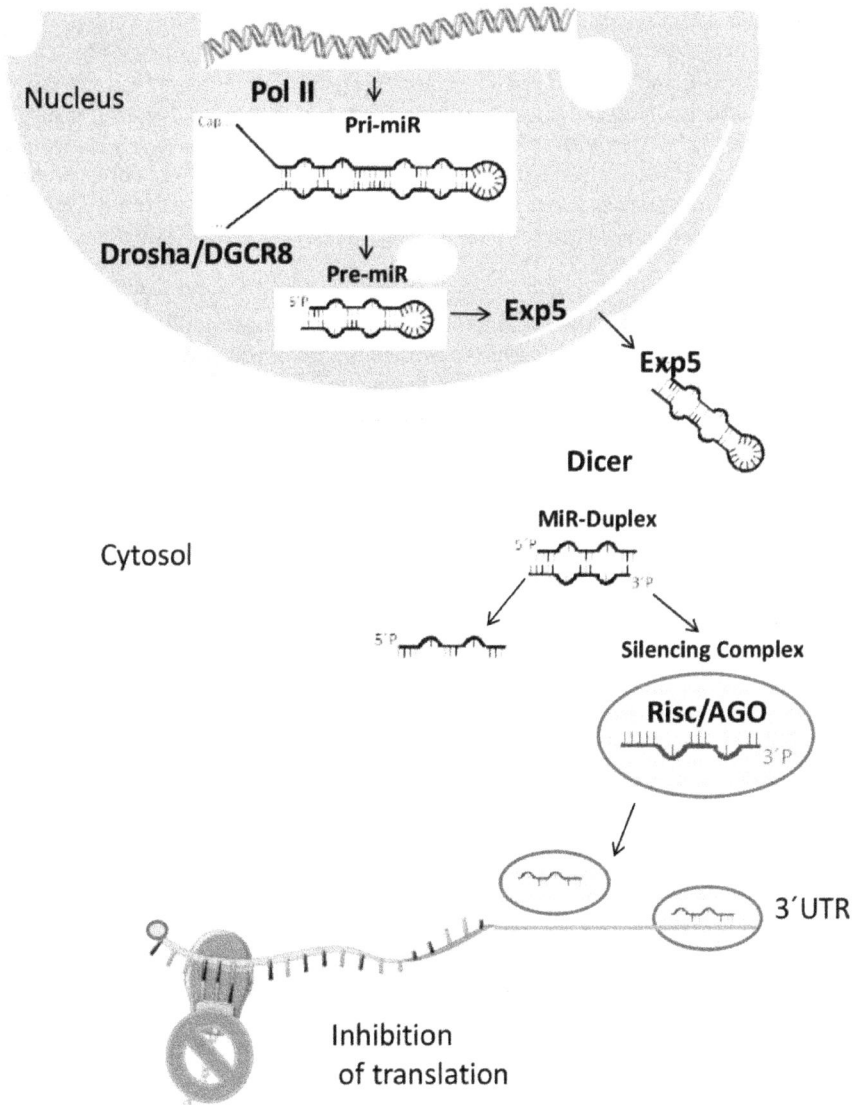

Figure 1.
Canonical pathway of biogenesis of miRs [31]. https://smart.servier.com/image-set-download/.

4. microRNAs and cancer

The miRs play a key role in the control of various physiological and pathological processes. Many studies demonstrate the participation of miRs during the progression of several types of cancer. MiRs present altered expression in tumors, and many studies are being conducted with this new class of molecules to elucidate their role in controlling the pathophysiology of the disease [36, 38, 39].

There is evidence that miRs are also involved in regulation of hallmarks of cancer and thus in the progression of cancer [5, 15]. In view of this, there is an effort by the scientific community to understand the mechanisms involving miRs and the development of cancer aiming to develop cancer-specific gene therapies [40]. The aim of these efforts is to improve responses to conventional drugs for the cancer treatment, specifically suppress oncogenic processes, and improve the prognosis of the disease.

The *miR-124* was one of the first studied miRs involved in the pathogenesis of cancer [41]. *MiR-124* was silenced in more than 10 types of cancer, as breast, colorectal, liver, and lung cancer. This silencing promotes increased expression of *CDK6*, which affects the phosphorylation state of *Rb* protein, favoring tumor progression [42]. Other miRs silenced are *miR-9-1* and *miR-9-3*. When analyzing the expression of *miR-9-3* in primary and metastatic tumors, it was observed that metastatic tumors have a lower expression of *miR-9-3*. Also, patients with lower *miR-9-3* expression in the tumor have a lower survival rate than patients with higher expression of *miR-9-3* [43].

Garzon et al. [40] observed that there is a decrease in *miRs-15a/16* expression in patients with chronic lymphoid leukemia and in chronic lymphocytic leukemia tumor cells CLL23. Thus, the authors ectopically increased the expression of *miRs-15a/16* in CLL23 tumor cells and investigated the processes of proliferation and apoptosis. It was observed that with the increase of *miRs-15a/16* expression in CLL23 tumor cells, there is a higher apoptosis and less cellular proliferation. This response occurs because *miRs-15a/16* target *BCL-2* protein, an important antiapoptotic factor. *BCL-2* is known to be increased in tumors of cancer patients [40].

Moreover, *miR-34* has been shown to be downregulated in pancreatic cancer. The overexpression of *miR-34* in these cells increases apoptosis and inhibition of autophagy, reducing tumor growth [44]. Another example is the miR *Let-7* family, which targets *HRAS* and *HMGA2* as well as participates in the regulation of proliferation and cell cycle. *Let-7* family members are also negatively regulated in various types of cancers, and their overexpression results in inhibition of tumor growth in different cancer models [45, 46]. This is due to the fact that *Let-7* targets the major components of cell cycle progression, such as *KRAS*, *CCDN1*, *CDC34*, *HMGA2*, *E2F2*, and *Lin28* [45, 46].

In contrast, miRs may also be increased in cancer and their biological effects may potentiate the development of the disease. For example, the case of *miR-21* has a high expression in tumors of glioblastoma, pancreatic cancer, breast cancer, and colon cancer. Inhibition of *miR-21* in glioblastoma cells was able to increase caspase activity and promote apoptosis of tumor cells. One possible explanation is that *miR-21* targets *PTEN* protein and *PDCD4* protein, functioning as an antiapoptotic agent in cancer [47].

MiRs are also involved in several other cancer factors, such as in the formation of metastases. Zhou et al. [48] observed that *miR-105* is involved with preparation of the "premetastatic niche." The authors demonstrated that animals with breast cancer exhibit high levels of *miR-105* expression in both tumor and circulation and that elevated *miR-105* levels in the circulation promote the destruction of endothelial barriers and increase vascular permeability in the target metastatic organ. Inhibition of *miR-105* in tumor cells from highly metastatic breast cancer prevented the development of metastasis [48]. Another miR associated with metastasis formation is the family of *miR-200*. The 200 family plays a role in repress proteins that promote the epithelial-mesenchymal transition. However, its expression is reduced in tumors in response to increased expression of the *long noncoding RNA ATB* that competes with the miRs binding site of the 200 family, reducing its expression and function, which favors the negative regulation of *E-cadherin* and increase of *ZEB* proteins expression [49]. The current involvement of miRs in the hallmarks of cancer is elucidated in **Figure 2**.

4.1 Physical activity as nonpharmacological therapy

Although in recent time cancer treatments have evolved considerably, there are still no responsive patients to the treatments, which suggest the need for strategies to reduce the incidence and aggressiveness of cancer. At same time, *American Cancer Society* recommends to cancer survivors the participation in 150 min of moderate intensity exercise per week. There is evidence that physical activity improves quality of life, treatment response, decreases cancer recurrence due physical fitness improvement of patients, and survivors [50]. In the present moment, there is strong academic effort in clinical trials being performed, investigating about perspective and limitation of inclusion physical activities in the cancer therapy. The main investigations focus in physiological aspects and appropriate modalities and methods [51–53].

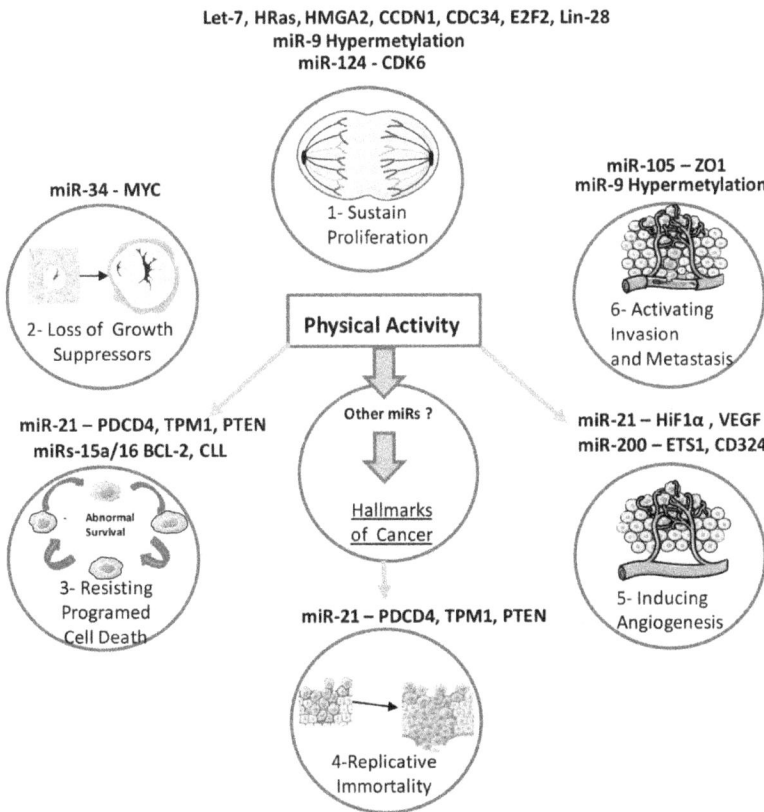

Figure 2.
Landscape of investigative field involving miRs, molecular basis, and the hallmarks of cancer. Currently, among the miRs related to the cancer hallmarks, only miR-21 and its target, the mRNA of PDCD4, PTEN, TPM1, HIF1α and VEGF was established the beneficial relationship with the effects of physical activity in the tumor (thin green arrows) [43–49, 83, 84]. https://smart.servier.com/image-set-download/.

Physical fitness is the ability to perform daily tasks with vigor and alertness, without excessive fatigue and with energy to enjoy leisure activities and to meet unforeseen emergencies [54]. It is known that physical activity induces beneficial adaptations to the body, improving physical fitness [55]. Physical activity encompasses both physical exercise with controlled volume, intensity, and duration or recreational activities [56]. There is evidence that support the importance of maintaining a physically active life for health. Healthy individuals or cardiovascular patients who have low physical capacity tend to have a lower survival rate [57]. Corroborating with these clinical and epidemiological data, experimental results show that rats with high capacity to run present a higher survival (~45%) when compared to those that have low capacity to run [58, 59]. Regular physical activities are recognized as nonpharmacologic preventive approach and treatment for chronic diseases [60–62], including cancer [63–65]. Several studies also demonstrate that aerobic physical activity normalizes the expression of aberrant miRs due to diseases such as myocardial infarction, hypertension, diabetes, and obesity. That these pathologies induce molecular and structural alterations and aerobic physical exercise is a beneficial stimulus for the reversal and control of these deleterious alterations such as muscle mass decrease and microvascular rarefaction [66–69].

4.2 Physical activity, cancer, and microRNAs: new perspectives

There is evidence that aerobic physical activity reduces the incidence of several types of cancer [65]. Moore et al. [65] demonstrated that regular physical activity resulted in decreased incidence of 13 types of cancer in 26 analyzed in 1.44 million adults. The individuals involved with higher daily volumes of physical activity presented decrease in the incidence in esophageal adenocarcinoma, myeloid leukemia, myeloma, liver, lung, kidney, gastric, endometrial, colon, head and neck, rectal, bladder, and breast cancer. The effects of physical activity on reducing the incidence of cancer were independent of other factors such as body mass index (BMI), smoking, geographical region, use of hormonal therapy, and ethnicity [65]. Cancer patients with reduced physical capacity have a worse prognosis [70–72]. Colon cancer patients have a reduction of more than 20% in maximal oxygen consumption (VO_2 máx.) compared to their healthy peers [71]. Patients with lung cancer and colon cancer with greater physical capacity present a higher survival compared to patients with lower physical capacity [73]. Aerobic physical activity attenuates tumor growth in different animal models [74–78]. However, the molecular mechanisms involved in this response are poorly understood. Recently, Pedersen et al. [79] showed that 4 weeks of prior voluntary physical activity was able to delay tumor initiation and attenuate tumor growth in various cancer models in mice and was also efficient in decreasing the formation of metastatic nodules. The authors demonstrated that physical activity increases the mobilization and redistribution of NK cells to the tumor microenvironment due to the systemic increase of IL-6 and epinephrine induced by physical activity. This increase of immune response in the tumor microenvironment was proposed as the main mechanism induced by aerobic physical activity for the attenuation of tumor growth [79]. Betof et al. [77] also demonstrated that previous aerobic physical activity is capable of attenuating tumor growth in the 4T1 breast cancer model. The authors demonstrated that aerobic physical activity increased the pericytic coverage of tumor vessels and apoptosis of tumor cells, provided a greater functional neo-vascularization on the tumor endothelium, and consequently reduced the hypoxia regions in the tumor microenvironment [77]. Pigna et al. demonstrated that aerobic physical activity is also efficient in increasing the survival of animals injected with C26 (colon cancer) tumor cells lineages [80].

However, it is important to note that only two of the studies that observed attenuation of tumor growth induced by aerobic physical activity investigated the role of miR in this response, both in mice breast cancer injected with MC4-L2. Khori et al. observed that aerobic physical activity was efficient in reducing *miR-21* gene expression in animal tumors, inhibiting proliferation and migration of tumor cells. In addition, the *miR-21* downregulation was associated with increase of gene and protein *PDCD4* expression and *TPM1*, two tumor suppressor genes [81]. Isanejad et al. [82] also demonstrated that aerobic physical activity reduces tumor growth and increased the gene expression levels of *miRs-206* and *let-7* in the mammary tumor. Moreover, exercise-increased expression of *miR-206* and *let-7* decreased in the levels of gene expression of *HIF-1α*, *CD31*, and *VEGF* in mice, suggesting an anti-angiogenic effect, which contributed to the decrease of tumor angiogenesis and growth [82]. Both Khori et al. and Isanejad et al. observed involvement of miRs in the aerobic physical activity response, which enhanced the effects of treatment with tamoxifen and letrozole, respectively, on tumor growth and molecular responses [81, 82].

These results indicate the potential of physical activity in modulating the decompensated miRs in the tumor. Also, we can point to the potential of physical activity to an improved miRs profile in the tumor, and their direct role in the reduction of the tumor growth and aggressiveness. However, currently there is a gap in elucidating about the global molecular mechanisms by which physical activity induces the phenotypical improvement. Therefore, the interaction between cancer, miRs and the effect of physical activity in the several cancer types is a promisor field of investigation that certainly will develop a lot of knowledge about preventive, therapeutic, as well as the mechanisms by which physical activity acts is cancer.

5. Cancer cachexia

Cancer cachexia (CC) is a multifactorial syndrome characterized by continuous loss of muscle mass that can be conjugated or not by loss of fat mass. CC cannot be completely reversed by conventional nutritional support and leads to progressive functional disability [83]. The pathophysiology of CC is characterized by a negative protein balance, anorexia, and metabolic abnormalities [84]. CC individuals usually present with muscle weakness, asthenia and poor response to anticancer treatment, all of these processes contributes to patient mortality [85, 86].

Muscle atrophy in CC results from the imbalance in protein turnover due to exacerbated proteolytic activation, reduction of protein synthesis pathways, and reduced regenerative capacity in skeletal muscle [87, 88].

In this context, it is essential to understand the role of epigenetic factors in the loss of muscle mass in CC. There is massive evidence that epigenetic factors, for example histone acetylation, DNA methylation and miRs orchestrate processes such as muscle proliferation and differentiation, as well as skeletal muscle regenerative capacity [89–92]. To elucidate about the epigenetic factors that lead to the loss of muscle mass in CC also may contribute to the emergence of new therapies for the prevention and treatment of the syndrome.

In this section, we will approach about the role of miRs in the regulation of muscular trophism. Skeletal muscle presents a set of miRs that are enriched in this tissue and mediate mechanisms of proliferation, differentiation, and protein synthesis. These miRs are known as myomiRs [32]. The most studied myomiRs are the *-133a/b*, *−206*, and *−1 miRs*. These miRs are known to display target genes such as *IGF-1R*, known hypertrophic pathway promoters [32] and *PAX3* and *PAX7*, genes that regulates proliferation of satellite cells [93]. In another view, there are many studies showing the role of several other miRs orchestrating prohypertrophic and procatabolic genes in the skeletal muscle [32, 94].

Interesting advances have been made in studies about the of role skeletal muscle enriched miRs in CC. Lee et al. [95] conducted a study in order to investigate the profile of miRs expressed in skeletal muscle of cachectic mice. The researchers performed a sequencing of the anterior tibial muscle of LLC tumor-bearing mice, animal model of orthotopic lung cancer, and compared them to healthy mice. The *miRs-147-3p*, *−299a-3p*, *1933-3p*, *511-3p*, *3473d*, *233-3p*, *431-5p*, *665-3p*, and *205-3p* were found to be differently expressed. Genetic ontology analyzes of these miRs indicate a relationship with cellular survival pathways, inflammatory response, cell cycle, cell development, and cell morphology through crosstalk of several pathways, with target genes such as *FOXO3*, *HRAS*, *P38*, *MAPK*, *MYC,* and *EIF4E*. We can note that *HRAS* and *MYC* are also related to hallmarks of cancer [95].

Narasimhan et al. [96] conducted another study evaluating the profile of miRs in muscle tissue of CC patients. In this study, human rectal abdominal muscle samples were collected during the tumor resection surgery of colon and pancreatic cancer patients. Sequencing analyzes demonstrated that eight miRs were differentially expressed between cachectic individuals and controls. The miRs let-*7d-3p*, *3184-3p*, and *−1296-5p* were selected and these miRs were increased in cachectic patients relative to controls. The authors performed *in-silico* analyzes and pointed out that these miRs targets genes related to adipogenesis, myogenesis (*SULF1* and *DLK1*), inflammation, and immune response (*RPS6KA6*) [96].

The loss of fat mass is not present in all cases of CC; however, the role in energy metabolism of adipose tissue in CC is important. Therefore, studies are being conducted to understand the function of miRs in maintaining of adipose tissue in cachetic state. Kulyté et al. [97] conducted a sequencing analyzes of miRs in adipose tissue of cachectic and noncachectic gastrointestinal cancer patients, the authors found difference in expression of nine miRs between cachectic and noncachectic patients. *MiR-378* was selected due to an increased expression in the adipose tissue of cachectic patients compared to noncachectic patients. The inhibition and overexpression of *miR-378* on human adipose-derived stem cells were performed; overexpression of *miR-378* decreased expression of the *HSL*, *PLIN1*, and *ATGL* protein and consequently increased lipids catabolism and release of glycerol [97].

MiRs are also present in body fluids such as saliva, tear, and blood. In this sense, studies are being conducted with the purpose of understanding the role of circulating miRs in CC. Okugawa et al. [98] showed that the expression of circulating *miR-21* increases in the patients with cachectic colon cancer; however, the expression of *miR-21* is not different in the skeletal muscle in compared to noncachectic patients [98]. The circulating miRs can be studied as biomarkers for some pathological processes. Studies in humans and animals have looked for miRs that are biomarkers in order to early diagnose CC [94]; however, it should be noted that many of these miRs are not widely accepted as biomarkers by the medical and scientific community and some are not even validated in humans [96].

The role of *miR-21* in CC was also investigated by He et al. [99], which showed that *miR-21*-enriched exosomes were found in the circulation of pancreatic and lung cancer patients. Myoblast cells cultures treated with these *miR-21*-enriched exosomes showed an interaction of the microvesicle with the muscle cells that induced cell death via *TLR8* protein, an endosomal receptor that recognizes single-stranded RNA (ssRNA), and can recognize ssRNA viruses such as Influenza, Sendai, and Coxsackie B viruses. *TLR8* is a protein binding to RNA and is able to recruit *MYD88* and leads to activation of the transcription factor *NF-κB* and an antiviral response. *TLR8* agonists have undergone clinical trials as immune stimulants in combination therapy for some cancers [99].

There are few studies showing a direct association of the action of miRs and their targets about processes involved in the progression or reversal of CC. The issue promises a great field for development of results that can be clinically relevant and useful in the future. Additionally, skeletal muscle is highly responsive to both physical activity and CC, and investigation of skeletal muscle-enriched miRs and the effect of physical activity and exercise in these miRs are promising to elucidate about CC. The next section will cover this topic.

5.1 Relationship between physical exercise and the mediators of cachexia

There is massive evidence that support the importance of maintaining aerobic fitness for health. Low aerobic fitness is an independent indicator of early death in individuals with cardiovascular and/or healthy individuals [57]. The physical training regulates the expression of miRs in a profile that enables endurance performance and physical fitness. Aerobic exercise prevents a number of chronic-degenerative diseases [60], including cancer [65]. Resistance training increases muscle mass and strength and contributes to increased functional capacity [87]. Therefore, aerobic and resistance training are presented as a therapeutic potential for CC patients and presents an interesting field of investigation to clarify clinically relevant process related to CC. However, due to clinical difficulties and poor safety conditions, there is a lack in human studies about the role of physical exercise in CC patients. In this context, the use of animal models in well-controlled studies has shown that physical training may be promising in the treatment of CC. Oh et al. demonstrated that the C26, orthotopic colon cancer cachectic mice, when submitted to resistance training and aerobic training protocols presented lower muscle mass loss [100]. Partial preservation of muscle mass due to physical training is associated with higher expression of proteins such as *mTOR*, *IGF*, and *myogenin* in the trained C26 mice when compared to sedentary C26 mice [100]. Pigna et al. demonstrated that voluntary aerobic activity in C26 mice also improves the autophagy flow preventing skeletal muscle loss in association with autophagy regulatory drugs [80]. Baggish et al. showed for the first time that *miRs-21*, *miR-146a*, and *-133a* are candidates to be biomarkers of aerobic physical training in the circulation [101].

Skeletal muscle trophism is regulated by the action of some miRs, and exercise controls the expression of these miRs. As example, *IGF-IR* mRNA encodes *IGF1* receptor protein and is a target of *miR-133*. A study shows that *IGF-IR* overexpression results in increased PI3K-AKT-mTOR pathway that mediated muscle hypertrophy, in myocyte cell culture, and that knockdown of *IGF-IR* decreases the hypertrophic signal. *MiR-133* decreases the expression of *IGF-IR*, and consequently decreases *AKT* and *mTOR* phosphorylation, regulating the development of skeletal muscle [102]. Furthermore, aerobic physical exercise decreases the expression of *miR-133a* [103].

In conclusion, many studies show that both aerobic and resistance physical exercise control the expression of miRs that are dysregulated by diseases as hypertension, diabetes, and obesity [68, 69, 104, 105]. Physical exercise rebalances the expression of the miRs involved with those alterations reverses structural deleterious changes in the skeletal muscle and restores tissue or prevents deterioration [66]. However, there are no studies designing an miR profile from CC skeletal muscle and the prevention of muscle catabolism by physical exercise, which is interesting for future investigation.

6. Conclusions

The effects of physical activity as nonpharmacological adjuvant for cancer patients are effective to the disease and survivorship in cancer, since it improves quality of life and decreases the recurrence of cancer. Currently, there are massive efforts to include exercise in the therapeutic approach to patients. Furthermore, studies show several benefits of aerobic physical activity in reducing the risk of incidence of cancer. Physical activity also reduces expenditures for public health agencies, both by decrease of cancer incidence and can attenuate the side effects or resistance related to anticancer treatment. However, little is known about the epigenetic, molecular, and cellular mechanisms involved in this response, both related to hallmarks of cancer, to cachexia process, and the comprehension about physical training effect in oncologic patients remains incipient.

Recently, the attentions of several areas of the scientific community have turned to miRs, epigenetic regulators in different cellular processes, as in tumorigenesis. To date, studies postulating the effects of aerobic physical activity on the modulation of decompensated miRNAs in the tumor and its potential as cancer gene therapy in cancer are rare. Thus, the identification of miRs modified by cancer of sedentary animals in comparison with trained animals can lead to the identification of miRs with therapeutic potential and elucidate about epigenetic mechanisms involved in physical activity therapy. However, it is necessary to better understand these mechanisms both in cell culture and in animal models of cancer in order to transpose into translational medicine in a whole approach. In this sense, extensive basic research is needed to elucidate these mechanisms in order to establish relationships about the role of miRs, the 10 biological capacities, the hallmarks of cancer, and if how these processes can be reversed by physical activity. Another interesting issue to be investigated is about the involvement of the miRs regulated by the physical activity in the CC and how these miRs are related to the 10 capacities and the hallmarks of cancer. These approaches can extensively clarify about cancer mechanisms and improve future physical activity therapy.

Acknowledgements

The researchers were supported by Sao Paulo Research Foundation (FAPESP: 2015/22814-5, 2015/17275-8, 2015/09919-2, 2017/22069-3, and 2018/02351-9), USP/PRP-NAPmiR, National Council for Scientific and Technological Development (CNPq: 307591/2009-3, 159827/2011-6, and 313479/2017-8), and Coordination for the Improvement of Higher Education Personnel (CAPES-Proex).

Conflict of interest

No disclosures.

Abbreviations

3'UTR region	3' untranslated region
AKT	AKT serine/threonine kinase
AGO	argonaute protein
ATGL	patatin-like phospholipase domain-containing protein 2
BCL2	B-cell lymphoma 2
BMI	body mass index
CC	cancer cachexia
CCDN1	cyclin D1

CD324	cadherin 1
CDC34	cell division cycle 34
CDK6	cell division protein kinase 6
DGCR8	DiGeorge syndrome critical region gene 8 microprocessor protein
DLK1	delta like non-canonical Notch ligand 1
DNA	deoxyribonucleic acid
E2F2	E2F transcription factor 2
EIF4E	eukaryotic translation initiation factor 4E
EMT	epithelial-mesenchymal transition
ETS1	ETS proto-oncogene 1
FOXO3	forkhead box O3
HDL	high-density lipoprotein
HiF1α	hypoxia inducible factor 1 alpha
HMGA2	high-mobility group AT-hook 2
HRAS	HRas proto-oncogene
HSL	hormone-sensitive lipase
IGF	insulin-like growth factor
IGF-1R	insulin like growth factor 1 receptor
IL-6	interleukin 6
MAPK	mitogen-activated protein kinase
VO$_{2máx}$	maximal oxygen consumption
mRNA	messenger RNA
miR	microRNA
mTOR	mechanistic target of rapamycin kinase
MYC	Myc proto-oncogene
MyD88	myeloid differentiation primary response
NK cells	natural killer cells
P38	mitogen-activated protein kinase 14
PAX3	paired box 3
PAX7	paired box 7
PDCD4	programmed cell death protein 4
PTEN	phosphatase and tensin homolog
PIK3CA	phosphatidylinositol-4,5-bisphosphate 3-kinase catalytic subunit alpha
PI3K	phosphatidylinositol-4,5-bisphosphate 3-kinase
PLIN1	perilipin 1
PDCD4	programmed cell death 4
RISC	RNA induced silencer complex
RPS6KA6	ribosomal protein S6 kinase A6
SULF1	sulfatase 1
TLR8	toll like receptor 8
TPM1	tropomyosin 1
VEGF	vascular endothelial growth factor
ZO1	tight junction protein 1

Author details

Gabriel Cardial Tobias, João Lucas Penteado Gomes, Ursula Paula Renó Soci,
Tiago Fernandes and Edilamar Menezes de Oliveira*
School of Physical Education and Sport, University of Sao Paulo, Sao Paulo, Brazil

*Address all correspondence to: edilamar@usp.br

IntechOpen

References

[1] Miller KD, Siegel RL, Lin CC, Mariotto AB, Kramer JL, Rowland JH, et al. Cancer treatment and survivorship statistics, 2016. CA: A Cancer Journal for Clinicians. 2016;**66**(4):271-289

[2] Torre LA, Bray F, Siegel RL, Ferlay J, Lortet-tieulent J, Jemal A. Global Cancer Statistics, 2012. CA: A Cancer Journal for Clinicians. 2015;**65**(2):87-108

[3] Pestka S, Krause CD, Walter MR. Interferons, interferon-like cytokines, and their receptors. Immunological Reviews. 2004;**202**:8-32

[4] Chammas R. Câncer e o microambiente tumoral [Cancer and the Tumor Microenvironment]. Revista Médica (Puebla). 2010;**89**(1):21-31

[5] Hanahan D, Weinberg RA. Hallmarks of cancer: The next generation. Cell. 2011;**144**(5):646-674

[6] Hanahan D, Weinbreg. The hallmarks of cancer. Cell Press. 2000;**100**(7):57-70

[7] Tisdale MJ. Reversing cachexia. Cell. 2010;**142**(4):511-512

[8] Moses AWG, Slater C, Preston T, Barber MD, Fearon KCH. Reduced total energy expenditure and physical activity in cachectic patients with pancreatic cancer can be modulated by an energy and protein dense oral supplement enriched with n-3 fatty acids. British Journal of Cancer. 2004;**90**(5):996-1002

[9] Bachmann J, Heiligensetzer M, Krakowski-Roosen H, Büchler MW, Friess H, Martignoni ME. Cachexia worsens prognosis in patients with resectable pancreatic cancer. Journal of Gastrointestinal Surgery. 2008;**12**(7):1193-1201

[10] Fearon KC, Voss AC, Hustead DS. Definition of cancer cachexia: Effect of weight loss, reduced food intake, and systemic inflammation on functional status and prognosis. The American Journal of Clinical Nutrition. 2006;**83**(6):1345-1350

[11] Anderson WF, Rosenberg PS, Prat A, Perou CM, Sherman ME. How many etiological subtypes of breast cancer: Two, three, four, or more? Journal of the National Cancer Institute. 2014;**106**(8):1-11

[12] Lago CU, Sung HJ, Ma W, Wang P, Hwang PM. P53, aerobic metabolism, and cancer. Antioxidants & Redox Signaling. 2011;**15**(6):1739-1748

[13] Waning DL, Mohammad KS, Reiken S, Xie W, Andersson DC, John S, et al. Excess TGF-β mediates muscle weakness associated with bone metastases in mice. Nature Medicine. 2015;**21**(11):1262-1271

[14] Peinado H, Alečković M, Lavotshkin S, Matei I, Costa-Silva B, Moreno-Bueno G, et al. Melanoma exosomes educate bone marrow progenitor cells toward a pro-metastatic phenotype through MET. Nature Medicine. 2012;**18**(6):883-891

[15] Yuan J, Yang F, Wang F, Ma J, Guo Y, Tao Q, et al. A long noncoding RNA activated by TGF-β promotes the invasion-metastasis cascade in hepatocellular carcinoma. Cancer Cell. 2014;**25**(5):666-681

[16] Kaplan RN, Riba RD, Zacharoulis S, Bramley AH, Vincent L, Costa C, et al. VEGFR1-positive haematopoietic bone marrow progenitors initiate the pre-metastatic niche. Nature. 2005;**438**(7069):820-827

[17] Pusapati RV, Daemen A, Wilson C, Sandoval W, Gao M, Haley B, et al. MTORC1-dependent metabolic reprogramming underlies escape from

glycolysis addiction in cancer cells. Cancer Cell. 2016;**29**(4):548-562

[18] Qu L, Ding J, Chen C, Wu ZJ, Liu B, Gao Y, et al. Exosome-transmitted lncARSR promotes sunitinib resistance in renal cancer by acting as a competing endogenous RNA. Cancer Cell. 2016;**29**(5):653-668

[19] Vazquez F, Lim JH, Chim H, Bhalla K, Girnun G, Pierce K, et al. PGC1α expression defines a subset of human melanoma tumors with increased mitochondrial capacity and resistance to oxidative stress. Cancer Cell. 2013;**23**(3):287-301

[20] Luo C, Lim JH, Lee Y, Granter SR, Thomas A, Vazquez F, et al. A PGC1α-mediated transcriptional axis suppresses melanoma metastasis. Nature. 2016;**537**(7620):422-426

[21] Lim JH, Luo C, Vazquez F, Puigserver P. Targeting mitochondrial oxidative metabolism in melanoma causes metabolic compensation through glucose and glutamine utilization. Cancer Research. 2014;**74**(13):3535-3545

[22] Choi W, Porten S, Kim S, Willis D, Plimack ER, Hoffman-Censits J, et al. Identification of distinct basal and luminal subtypes of muscle-invasive bladder cancer with different sensitivities to frontline chemotherapy. Cancer Cell. 2014;**25**(2):152-165

[23] Lu F, Chen Y, Zhao C, Wang H, He D, Xu L, et al. Olig2-dependent reciprocal shift in PDGF and EGF receptor signaling regulates tumor phenotype and mitotic growth in malignant glioma. Cancer Cell. 2016;**29**(5):669-683

[24] Peinado H, Zhang H, Matei IR, Costa-Silva B, Hoshino A, Rodrigues G, et al. Pre-metastatic niches: Organ-specific homes for metastases. Nature Reviews Cancer. 2017

[25] Nebbioso A, Tambaro FP, Dell'Aversana C, Altucci L. Cancer epigenetics: Moving forward. PLoS Genetics. 2018;**14**(6):1-25

[26] Flavahan WA, Gaskell E, Bernstein BE. Epigenetic plasticity and the hallmarks of cancer. Science (80-). 2017;**357**(6348)

[27] Murtha M, Esteller M. Extraordinary cancer epigenomics: Thinking outside the classical coding and promoter box. Trends in Cancer. 2016;**2**(10):572-584

[28] Berger SL, Kouzarides T, Shiekhattar R, Shilatifard A. An operational definition of epigenetics. Genes & Development. 2009:23-25

[29] Muñoz-Pinedo C, González-Suárez E, Portela A, Gentilella A, Esteller M. Exploiting tumor vulnerabilities: Epigenetics, cancer metabolism and the mtor pathway in the era of personalized medicine. Cancer Research. 2013;**73**(14):4185-4189

[30] Bardhan K, Liu K. Epigenetics and colorectal cancer pathogenesis. Cancers (Basel). 2013;**5**(2):676-713

[31] Alderton GK. Tumour evolution: Epigenetic and genetic heterogeneity in metastasis. Nature Reviews. Cancer. 2017;**17**(3):141-141

[32] Horak M, Novak J, Bienertova-Vasku J. Muscle-specific microRNAs in skeletal muscle development. Developmental Biology. 2016;**410**(1):1-13

[33] Lee RC, Feinbaum RL, Ambros V. The *C. elegans* heterochronic gene lin-4 encodes small RNAs with antisense complementarity to lin-14. Cell. 1993;**75**(5):843-854

[34] Hong Y, Lee RC, Ambros V. Structure and function analysis of LIN-14, a temporal regulator of postembryonic developmental events in

Caenorhabditis elegans. Molecular and Cellular Biology. 2000;**20**(6):2285-2295

[35] Ambros V. microRNAs: Tiny regulators with great potential. Cell. 2001;**107**(7):823-826

[36] Bartel DP. Metazoan microRNAs. Cell [Internet]. 2018;**173**(1):20-51. DOI: 10.1016/j.cell.2018.03.006

[37] Creemers EE, Tijsen AJ, Pinto YM. Circulating MicroRNAs. Circulation Research. 2012;**110**(3):483-495

[38] Müller S, Nowak K. Exploring the miRNA-mRNA regulatory network in clear cell renal cell carcinomas by next-generation sequencing expression profiles. BioMed Research International. 2014;**2014**(948408):1-11

[39] Tutar Y. miRNA and cancer; computational and experimental approaches. Current Pharmaceutical Biotechnology. 2014;**15**(5):429

[40] Garzon R, Marcucci G, Croce CM. Targeting microRNAs in cancer: Rationale, strategies and challenges. Nature Reviews Clinical Oncology. 2010;**48**(Suppl 2):1-6

[41] Lujambio A, Ropero S, Ballestar E, Fraga MF, Cerrato C, Setien F, et al. Genetic unmasking of an epigenetically silenced microRNA in human cancer cells. Cancer Research. 2007;**67**(4):1424-1429

[42] Baer C, Claus R, Plass C. Genome-wide epigenetic regulation of miRNAs in cancer. Cancer Research. 2013;**73**(2):473-477

[43] Hildebrandt MAT, Gu J, Lin J, Ye Y, Tan W, Tamboli P, et al. Hsa-miR-9 methylation status is associated with cancer development and metastatic recurrence in patients with clear cell renal cell carcinoma. Oncogene. 2010;**29**(42):5724-5728

[44] Gibori H, Eliyahu S, Krivitsky A, Ben-Shushan D, Epshtein Y, Tiram G, et al. Amphiphilic nanocarrier-induced modulation of PLK1 and MIR-34a leads to improved therapeutic response in pancreatic cancer. Nature Communications. 2018;**9**(1)

[45] Brueckner B, Stresemann C, Kuner R, Mund C, Musch T, Meister M, et al. The human let-7a-3 locus contains an epigenetically regulated microRNA gene with oncogenic function. Cancer Research. 2007;**67**(4):1419-1423

[46] Wang T, Wang G, Hao D, Liu X, Wang D, Ning N, et al. Aberrant regulation of the LIN28A/LIN28B and let-7 loop in human malignant tumors and its effects on the hallmarks of cancer. Molecular Cancer. 2015;**14**(1):1-13

[47] Chan JA, Krichevsky AM, Kosik KS. MicroRNA-21 is an antiapoptotic factor in human glioblastoma cells. Cancer Research. 2005;**65**(14):6029-6033

[48] Zhou W, Fong MY, Min Y, Somlo G, Liu L, Palomares MR, et al. Cancer-secreted miR-105 destroys vascular endothelial barriers to promote metastasis. Cancer Cell. 2014;**25**(4):501-515

[49] Chan YC, Khanna S, Roy S, Sen CK. MiR-200b targets Ets-1 and is down-regulated by hypoxia to induce angiogenic response of endothelial cells. The Journal of Biological Chemistry. 2011;**286**(3):2047-2056

[50] Rock CL, Doyle C, Demark-Wahnefried W, Meyerhardt J, Courneya KS, Schwartz AL, et al. Nutrition and physical activity guidelines for cancer survivors. CA: A Cancer Journal for Cinicians. 2012;**62**(2):242-274

[51] Alibhai SMH, Santa Mina D, Ritvo P, Sabiston C, Krahn M, Tomlinson G, et al. A phase II RCT and economic

analysis of three exercise delivery methods in men with prostate cancer on androgen deprivation therapy. BMC Cancer. 2015

[52] Segal RJ, Reid RD, Courneya KS, Sigal RJ, Kenny GP, Prud'Homme DG, et al. Randomized controlled trial of resistance or aerobic exercise in men receiving radiation therapy for prostate cancer. Journal of Clinical Oncology. 2009;**27**(3):344-351

[53] Newton RU, Taaffe DR, Spry N, Gardiner RA, Levin G, Wall B, et al. A phase III clinical trial of exercise modalities on treatment side-effects in men receiving therapy for prostate cancer. BMC Cancer. 2009

[54] World Health Organization. Physical Activity [Internet]. 2017. Available from: http://www.who.int/topics/physical_activity/en/

[55] Egan B, Zierath JR. Exercise metabolism and the molecular regulation of skeletal muscle adaptation. Cell Metabolism. 2013;**17**(2):162-184

[56] Caspersen CJ, Powell KE, Christenson GM. Physical activity, exercise, and physical fitness: Definitions and distinctions for health-related research. Public Health Reports. 1985;**100**(2):126-131

[57] Kokkinos P, Myers J, Kokkinos JP, Pittaras A, Narayan P, Manolis A, et al. Exercise capacity and mortality in Black and White men. Circulation. 2008;**117**(5):614-622

[58] Koch LG, Kemi OJ, Qi N, Leng SX, Bijma P, Gilligan LJ, et al. Intrinsic aerobic capacity sets a divide for aging and longevity. Circulation Research. 2011;**109**(10):1162-1172

[59] Wisløff U, Najjar SM, Ellingsen Ø, Haram PM, Swoap S, Al-Share Q, et al. Cardiovascular risk factors emerge after artificial selection for low aerobic capacity. Science (80-). 2005;**307**(5708):418-420

[60] Pahor M, Guralnik JM, Ambrosius WT, Blair S, Bonds DE, Church TS, et al. Effect of structured physical activity on prevention of major mobility disability in older adults: The LIFE study randomized clinical trial. JAMA. 2014;**311**(23):2387-2396

[61] Fiuza-Luces C, Garatachea N, Berger NA, Lucia A. Exercise is the real polypill. Physiology. 2013;**28**(5):330-358

[62] Flachenecker P. Autoimmune diseases and rehabilitation. Autoimmunity Reviews. 2012;**11**(3): 219-225

[63] Neilson HK, Friedenreich CM, Brockton NT, Millikan RC. Physical activity and postmenopausal breast cancer: Proposed biologic mechanisms and areas for future research. Cancer Epidemiology, Biomarkers & Prevention. 2009;**18**(1):11-27

[64] Friedenreich CM, Cust AE. Physical activity and breast cancer risk: Impact of timing, type and dose of activity and population subgroup effects. British Journal of Sports Medicine. 2008;**42**(8):636-647

[65] Moore SC, Lee IM, Weiderpass E, Campbell PT, Sampson JN, Kitahara CM, et al. Association of leisure-time physical activity with risk of 26 types of cancer in 1.44 million adults. JAMA Internal Medicine. 2016;**176**(6):816-825

[66] Fernandes T, Magalhães FC, Roque FR, Phillips MI, Oliveira EM. Exercise training prevents the microvascular rarefaction in hypertension balancing angiogenic and apoptotic factors: Role of microRNAs-16, -21, and -126. Hypertension. 2012;**59**(2 SUPPL. 1): 513-520

[67] Melo SFS, Fernandes T, Baraúna VG, Matos KC, Santos AAS, Tucci PJF,

et al. Expression of microRNA-29 and collagen in cardiac muscle after swimming training in myocardial-infarcted rats. Cellular Physiology and Biochemistry. 2014;**33**(3):657-669

[68] Gomes JLP, Fernandes T, Soci UPR, Silveira AC, Barretti DLM, Negrão CE, et al. Obesity downregulates microRNA-126 inducing capillary rarefaction in skeletal muscle: Effects of aerobic exercise training. Oxidative Medicine and Cellular Longevity. 2017;**2017**

[69] Fernandes T, Casaes L, Soci U, Silveira A, Gomes J, Barretti D, et al. Exercise training restores the cardiac microrna-16 levels preventing microvascular rarefaction in obese Zucker rats. Obesity Facts. 2018;**11**(1)

[70] Koelwyn GJ, Jones LW, Moslehi J. Unravelling the causes of reduced peak oxygen consumption in patients with cancer: Complex, timely, and necessary. Journal of American College of Cardiology. 2014;**64**(13):1320-1322

[71] Cramer L, Hildebrandt B, Kung T, Wichmann K, Springer J, Doehner W, et al. Cardiovascular function and predictors of exercise capacity in patients with colorectal cancer. Journal of the American College of Cardiology. 2014;**64**(13):1310-1319

[72] Jones LW, Courneya KS, Mackey JR, Muss HB, Pituskin EN, Scott JM, et al. Cardiopulmonary function and age-related decline across the breast cancer: Survivorship continuum. Journal of Clinical Oncology. 2012;**30**(20):2530-2537

[73] Lakoski SG, Willis BL, Barlow CE, Leonard D, Gao A, Radford NB, et al. Midlife cardiorespiratory fitness, incident cancer, and survival after cancer in men: The Cooper Center Longitudinal Study. JAMA Oncology. 2015;**1**(2):231-237

[74] Goh J, Tsai J, Bammler TK, Farin FM, Endicott E, Ladiges WC. Exercise training in transgenic mice is associated with attenuation of early breast cancer growth in a dose-dependent manner. PLoS One. 2013;**8**(11):e80123

[75] Wolff G, Balke JE, Andras IE, Park M, Toborek M. Exercise modulates redox-sensitive small GTPase activity in the brain microvasculature in a model of brain metastasis formation. PLoS One. 2014;**9**(5):1-8

[76] Hojman P, Fjelbye J, Zerahn B, Christensen JF, Dethlefsen C, Lonkvist CK, et al. Voluntary exercise prevents cisplatin-induced muscle wasting during chemotherapy in mice. PLoS One. 2014;**9**(9):e109030

[77] Betof AS, Lascola CD, Weitzel D, Landon C, Scarbrough PM, Devi GR, et al. Modulation of murine breast tumor vascularity, hypoxia, and chemotherapeutic response by exercise. Journal of the National Cancer Institute. 2015;**107**(5):1-5

[78] Higgins KA, Park D, Lee GY, Curran WJ, Deng X. Exercise-induced lung cancer regression: Mechanistic findings from a mouse model. Cancer. 2014;**120**(21):3302-3310

[79] Pedersen L, Idorn M, Olofsson GH, Lauenborg B, Nookaew I, Hansen RH, et al. Voluntary running suppresses tumor growth through epinephrine- and IL-6-dependent NK cell mobilization and redistribution. Cell Metabolism. 2016;**23**(3):554-562

[80] Pigna E, Berardi E, Aulino P, Rizzuto E, Zampieri S, Carraro U, et al. Aerobic exercise and pharmacological treatments counteract cachexia by modulating autophagy in colon cancer. Scientific Reports. 2016;**6**(October 2015):26991

[81] Khori V, Amani Shalamzari S, Isanejad A, Alizadeh AM, Alizadeh S,

Khodayari S, et al. Effects of exercise training together with tamoxifen in reducing mammary tumor burden in mice: Possible underlying pathway of MIR-21. European Journal of Pharmacology. 2015;**765**:179-187

[82] Isanejad A, Alizadeh AM, Amani Shalamzari S, Khodayari H, Khodayari S, Khori V, et al. MicroRNA-206, let-7a and microRNA-21 pathways involved in the anti-angiogenesis effects of the interval exercise training and hormone therapy in breast cancer. Life Sciences. 2016;**151**:30-40

[83] Fearon K, Strasser F, Anker SD, Bosaeus I, Bruera E, Fainsinger RL, et al. Definition and classification of cancer cachexia: An international consensus. The Lancet Oncology. 2011;**12**(5):489-495

[84] Argilés JM, Busquets S, Stemmler B, López-Soriano FJ. Cancer cachexia: Understanding the molecular basis. Nature Reviews. Cancer. 2014;**14**(11):754-762

[85] Tisdale MJ. Mechanisms of cancer cachexia. Physiological Reviews. 2009;**89**(2):381-410

[86] Acunzo M, Croce CM. MicroRNA in cancer and cachexia—A mini-review. The Journal of Infectious Diseases. 2015;**212**(Suppl 1):S74-S77

[87] Schiaffino S, Dyar KA, Ciciliot S, Blaauw B, Sandri M. Mechanisms regulating skeletal muscle growth and atrophy. The FEBS Journal. 2013;**280**(17):4294-4314

[88] Fearon KCH, Glass DJ, Guttridge DC. Cancer cachexia: Mediators, signaling, and metabolic pathways. Cell Metabolism. 2012;**16**(2):153-166

[89] Segatto M, Fittipaldi R, Pin F, Sartori R, Ko KD, Zare H, et al. counteracts cancer cachexia and prolongs survival. Nature Communications:1-15

[90] Samant SA, Pillai VB, Gupta MP. Cellular mechanisms promoting cachexia and how they are opposed by sirtuins. Canadian Journal of Physiology and Pharmacology. 2018:1-38

[91] Fernandez-Zapico ME, Fernandez-Barrena MG, Marks DL. Discovering and targeting the epigenetic pathways to treat muscle loss: Working toward a paradigm shift in cancer therapeutics. Current Opinion in Supportive and Palliative Care. 2014:319-320

[92] Sharples AP, Polydorou I, Hughes DC, Owens DJ, Hughes TM, Stewart CE. Skeletal muscle cells possess a 'memory' of acute early life TNF-α exposure: Role of epigenetic adaptation. Biogerontology. 2016;**17**(3):603-617

[93] Dai Y, Wang YM, Zhang WR, Liu XF, Li X, Ding X, et al. The role of microRNA-1 and microRNA-206 in the proliferation and differentiation of bovine skeletal muscle satellite cells. In Vitro Cellular & Developmental Biology: Animal. 2016;**52**(1):27-34

[94] Siracusa J, Koulmann N, Banzet S. Circulating myomiRs: A new class of biomarkers to monitor skeletal muscle in physiology and medicine. Journal of Cachexia, Sarcopenia and Muscle. November;**2018**:20-27

[95] Lee DE, Brown JL, Rosa-Caldwell ME, Blackwell TA, Perry RA, Brown LA, et al. Cancer cachexia-induced muscle atrophy: Evidence for alterations in microRNAs important for muscle size. Physiological Genomics. 2018;**182**(16):253-260

[96] Narasimhan A, Ghosh S, Stretch C, Greiner R, Bathe OF, Baracos V, et al. Small RNAome profiling from human skeletal muscle: Novel miRNAs and their targets associated with cancer cachexia. January. 2017:405-416

[97] Kulyté A, Lorente-Cebrián S, Gao H, Mejhert N, Agustsson T, Arner P, et al.

MicroRNA profiling links miR-378 to enhanced adipocyte lipolysis in human cancer cachexia. American Journal of Physiology. Endocrinology and Metabolism. 2018:267-274

[98] Okugawa Y, Yao LI, Toiyama Y, Yamamoto A, Shigemori T, Yin C, et al. Prognostic impact of sarcopenia and its correlation with circulating miR-21 in colorectal cancer patients. Oncology Reports. 2018:1555-1564

[99] He WA, Calore F, Londhe P, Canella A, Guttridge DC, Croce CM. Microvesicles containing miRNAs promote muscle cell death in cancer cachexia via TLR7. Proceedings of the National Academy of Sciences of the United States of America. 2014;**111**(12):4525-4529

[100] Oh S, Elam ML, Jo E, Arjmandi BH. Aerobic and resistance training dependent skeletal muscle plasticity in the colon-26 murine model of cancer cachexia. Metabolism. 2016;**65**(5):685-698

[101] Baggish AL, Park J, Min P-K, Isaacs S, Parker BA, Thompson PD, et al. Rapid upregulation and clearance of distinct circulating microRNAs after prolonged aerobic exercise. Journal of Applied Physiology. 2014;**116**(5):522-531

[102] Yu H, Lu Y, Li Z, Wang Q. microRNA-133: Expression, function and therapeutic potential in muscle diseases and cancer. Current Drug Targets. 2014;**15**(9):817-828

[103] Safdar A, Saleem A, Tarnopolsky MA. The potential of endurance exercise-derived exosomes to treat metabolic diseases. Nature Reviews. Endocrinology. 2016;**12**(9):504-517

[104] Staszel T, Zapała B, Polus A, Sadakierska-Chudy A, Kieć-Wilk B, Stępień E, et al. Role of microRNAs in endothelial cell pathophysiology. Polskie Archiwum Medycyny Wewnętrznej. 2011;**121**(10):361-367

[105] Improta Caria AC, Nonaka CKV, Pereira CS, Soares MBP, Macambira SG, Souza BSF. Exercise training-induced changes in microRNAs: Beneficial regulatory effects in hypertension, type 2 diabetes, and obesity. International Journal of Molecular Sciences. 2018

Chapter 4

Consequences of Artificial Light at Night: The Linkage between Chasing Darkness Away and Epigenetic Modifications

Abraham Haim, Sinam Boynao and Abed Elsalam Zubidat

Abstract

Epigenetics is an important tool for understanding the relation between environmental exposures and cellular functions, including metabolic and proliferative responses. At our research center, we have devolved a mouse model for characterizing the relation between exposure to artificial light at night (ALAN) and both global DNA methylation (GDM) and breast cancer. Generally, the model describes a close association between ALAN and cancer responses. Cancer responses are eminent at all light spectra, with the prevalent manifestation at the shorter end of the visible spectrum. ALAN-induced pineal melatonin suppression is the principal candidate mechanism mediating the environmental exposure at the molecular level by eliciting aberrant GDM modifications. The carcinogenic potential of ALAN can be ameliorated in mice by exogenous melatonin treatment. In contrast to BALB/c mice, humans are diurnal species, and thus, it is of great interest to evaluate the ALAN-melatonin-GDM nexus also in a diurnal mouse model. The fat sand rat (*Psammomys obesus*) provides an appropriate model as its responses to photoperiod are comparable to humans. Interestingly, melatonin and thyroxin have opposite effects on GDM levels in *P. obesus*. Melatonin, GDM levels, and even thyroxin may be utilized as novel biomarkers for detection, staging, therapy, and prevention of breast cancer progression.

Keywords: melatonin, thyroxin, light-at-night, global DNA methylation, diurnal species, breast cancer, biomarkers

1. Introduction

Since the invention of electrical light in 1879 by Thomas Alva Edison, artificial light at night (ALAN) has become a definitive feature of human development with accelerated increase concurrent with urbanization and industrialization. The light emitted from the original bulb of Edison known as incandescent bulb was weak, with a dominant long wavelength emission above 560 nm. Most of the incandescent electrical energy is dissipated as heat energy, thus making this type of illumination energetically inefficient. Therefore, new illumination technologies were developed, in order to discover efficient bulbs that transfer most of the electrical energy into light. White fluorescent and light-emitting diodes (LED) are examples of energy efficient bulbs developed to decrease carbon dioxide production from electric power plants, thus lessening the greenhouse effect. One of the adverse outcomes of using efficient illumination at night time is the emission of shorter wavelengths (SWLs) that further exacerbate the health and ecological problems associated with a new source of environmental pollution currently known as ALAN [1–3]. Light pollution is increasing rapidly, resulting in a more illuminated world, where outdoor and indoor illumination sources are increasing ALAN in developed and developing countries [4, 5].

From an anthropological perspective, electric light has brought pronounced benefits including advancing urbanization and industrialization by increasing productivity, but we are also increasingly being aware of serious public health and ecological negative impacts emerging from disrupting the adaptive temporal organization of biological responses [6–8]. Certainly, multiple studies have shown the effects of light pollution on social, behavioral, physiological, and molecular responses in many different taxa, including insects [9], fishes [10], amphibians [11], reptiles [12], birds [13], and mammals [14], as well as plants [15]. Some of the most disturbing effects of ALAN on health are metabolic dysfunction and cancer progression [2, 16]. In mice and humans, several lines of evidence suggest a close association between ALAN levels and both obesity and breast cancer progression [17–19]. Here, we focus on ALAN as a novel environmental polluter that disrupts biological timing (temporal organization) and consequently may provoke severe health risk, particularly breast cancer development through epigenetic modifications. First, the mammalian photoperiodic system is reviewed in relation to light perception and downstream endocrine responses for timing biological rhythms. Thereafter, we discuss the sensitivity of the photoperiodic system to the spectral composition of ALAN, particularly SWL illuminations. We further discuss the ALAN signal transduction pathway involved in melatonin suppression and aberrant epigenetic modifications in breast cancer progression. Therefore, melatonin and epigenetics are suggested as new biomarkers for breast cancer prevention. Finally, melatonin and thyroxin treatments in the diurnal fat sand rat (*Psammomys obesus*) are discussed in relation to their potential role in mediating the environmental exposures at the molecular level *via* epigenetic modifications, particularly global DNA methylation (GDM).

2. The mammalian photoperiodic system

In an early study, it has been demonstrated that the blind mole rat (*Spalax ehrenbergi*) responded differently to short and long photoperiod manipulations in regard to its capability to cope with low ambient temperature exposure [20]. Results of a more recent study on *S. ehrenbergi* manifested robust and differential responses in metabolism, stress, and melatonin levels to ALAN of different spectral compositions and acclimation duration [21]. These results suggested that the vestigial retina of this species still expresses photoreceptors that are involved mainly in nonvisual response. Currently, the mammalian eye is described as a dual-function organ, expressing photoreceptors for both visual and nonvisual responses [22]. The visual response is mediated by two distinct photoreceptor types, rods and cones, which control scotopic vision and photopic vision, respectively [23]. The nonvisual responses are mainly mediated by intrinsically photosensitive retinal ganglion cells (ipRGCs) that express the photopigment melanopsin. Even though the ipRGCs are connected with rods and cones by bipolar cells, they mediate nonvisual responses including photo-entrainment of biological rhythms [24].

First, photoperiodic signals are perceived by ipRGCs that express the photo-pigment melanopsin [25]. The detected environmental light signal by the ipRGCs synchronizes the master circadian clock located in the mammalian hypothalamic suprachiasmatic nucleus (SCN) by the retinohypothalamic tract (RHT). The

SCN regulates the synthesis and release of the hormone melatonin by the pineal gland through multiunit sympathetic nerves from the superior cervical ganglion (SCG). The SCG presynaptic sympathetic terminals release noradrenalin that interacts with postsynaptic α- and β-adrenergic receptors to regulate synthesis and release of pineal melatonin [26]. In mammals, the activity of the adrenergic SCG terminals that innervate the pineal gland is stimulated by darkness and inhibited by light [27]. Under dark conditions, stimulation of the pineal adrenergic receptors increases cellular cAMP levels leading to the activation of aryl-alkyl-amine-N-acetyltransferase (AA-NAT), a key enzyme in melatonin synthesis [28]. The nocturnal increase in the enzymatic activity of AA-NAT is strongly inhibited by light exposure, consequently leading to a rapid decrease in nocturnal melatonin levels [29]. The pinealocytes are the primary neuroendocrine cells that synthesis melatonin by sequential hydroxylation and decarboxylation of its precursor tryptophan to serotonin. Thereafter, serotonin is acetylated by the rate-limiting enzyme AA-NAT and methylated by the enzyme hydroxyindole-O-methyltransferase (HIOMT) to the final product of melatonin [28, 30]. Finally, the activity of both AA-NAT and HIOMT is under photoperiodic control at the transcriptional level showing distinct diurnal rhythms with peak levels during night and nadir levels during the day [31].

3. Melatonin suppression as an indicator of SWL pollution

In most mammals, no level of light exposure is powerless regarding melatonin suppression and even low intensity and short-term exposures can reduce its production and lead to decreased circulating levels [32, 33]. Nonetheless, melatonin suppression is strongly wavelength- and irradiance-dependent, with faster and more robust response at the SWL end of the visible spectrum below 500 nm [19, 34, 35]. A large-scale study comparing the effect of different light technologies on melatonin production in humans demonstrated that the strongest suppression occurred in response to 4000 and 5000 K LED lights compared with incandescent, halogen, and fluorescent counterpart lightening systems [36]. Narrow bandwidth blue LED exposure (λ = 469 nm, ½ peak bandwidth = 26 nm) decreased melatonin levels in an irradiance dose-dependent manner, and this light was more effective in decreasing the hormone levels compared with that of 4000 K of white fluorescent at twice the energy of the latter [37]. In horses, 1 h exposure of 3 lux SWL blue light (468 nm) administered only to one eye was sufficient to decrease melatonin levels compared with control animals [38].

Furthermore, blue LED pulses (2-s pulse every 1 min for 1 h, λ = 450 nm) administrated through closed human eyelids markedly suppressed nocturnal melatonin levels and delayed the melatonin onset phase [39–41]. While the eyelids can weaken irradiance and wavelength ([42], light signals can still penetrate them, be detected by the retinal photoreceptors, and affect circadian regulation [43]. In humans, blue LED exposure (40 lux, 470 nm) emitted from display screens (tablets and computers), suppressed nocturnal melatonin in a duration-dependent manner [44, 45] and melatonin suppression showed higher sensitivity to wavelength compared with intensity manipulations [46].

Together, it is clear that the adverse effects of light pollution are strongly manifested by the SWL portion of the spectrum. As the LED illumination is becoming ubiquitous in every aspect of our modern life, the expected increase in light pollution may exacerbate the problem since higher irradiance and shorter wavelengths would be emitted by the energy efficient technology [47, 48]. Accordingly, the American Medical Association [49] passed a resolution in 2016 calling upon communities in the USA to avoid using LED lighting in public domains as it is enriched with SWL [49]. In summary, SWL-ALAN is a source of pollution and should be removed from public spaces through legislation.

4. ALAN as an environmental change and a model for studying epigenetic modifications

The flexibility and the sensitivity of the endocrine system play an adaptive role in determining the success and survival of organisms under contentiously changing environmental conditions in their habitat [50]. As the endocrine system regulates several functions, it is expected to be the first system to respond to environmental changes such as ALAN by coordinating body functions to maintain homeostasis during the exposure. The core stimulus-response of the endocrine system to ALAN relies on four main components, including the pineal gland, the hypothalamic-pituitary-gonadal (HPG) axis, the hypothalamic-pituitary-thyroid axis (HPT), and the hypothalamic-pituitary-adrenal (HPA) axis [51]. The elaborated hormonal responses generated by these axes to ALAN exposure might be mediated by transcriptional regulation of gene expression *via* epigenetic modifications [52]. Therefore, epigenetic-elicited alteration in gene expression is a potential transduction pathway by which hormonal responses (e.g., melatonin) may mediate environmental exposures (e.g., ALAN). Conversely, the ALAN-induced alteration in melatonin rhythms may also exert endocrine responses *via* epigenetic modifications [53].

The incidences of breast and prostate cancers show close association with light pollution particularly in urbanized and industrialized regions [2, 54]. Several epidemiological studies have found direct association between light pollution and incidence of breast cancer in women as well as prostate cancer in men [18, 55, 56]. Furthermore, the strong association between light pollution and cancer incidences displays divergent spatial disruption with higher incidences in urban compared with rural regions [57, 58]. Evidence for direct association between ALAN and cancer development comes also from animal studies.

In rats, ALAN exposure accelerated the growth rates of induced-tumors, including mammary cancer [59–62]. Studies under control conditions demonstrated that 30-min ALAN per midnight emitted from either white fluorescent or blue LED illuminations can accelerate tumor growth and lung metastatic activity in female BALB/c mice inoculated with 4T1 mammary carcinoma [63, 64]. Indeed, the effects of ALAN on tumor growth have been demonstrated at different spectral compositions with markedly higher cancer burden in response to lighting exposure lower than 500 nm [19].

These studies have related the increased cancer burden to aberrant epigenetic modifications, particularly advanced global DNA hypo-methylation. Promoter hyper-methylation of cancer suppresser genes and global DNA hypo-methylation are characterizing epigenetic patterns in breast cancer cells [65, 66]. These aberrant epigenetic modifications may contribute to increase cancer burden by eliciting genomic instability and activation of both oncogenes and metastatic related genes, as well as silencing tumor suppressor genes. Generally, prominent decreased methylation in repetitive DAN elements is a common trait in most cancer cells [67]. Demethylation of pro-metastatic genes is normally suppressed by DNA methylation and might advance gene overexpression leading to genetic instability that increases the risk of developing cancer [68, 69]. DNA hypomethylation can be detected at an early stage of breast cancer and is correlated with the degree of tumor differentiation [70, 71]. Altogether, the close association between aberrant

DAN hypomethylation and tumorigenesis, particularly of breast cancer, is well-established, but the underlying mechanism remains poorly understood, especially how the adverse ALAN effects are mediated.

5. Melatonin as a mediating signal linking ALAN and epigenetic-induced cancer

Since the melatonin hypothesis was first proposed during the late twentieth century by Stevens [72], multiple studies in human and nonhuman animals have provided direct and indirect evidence that melatonin suppression by ALAN could impose health risks, including metabolic disorders and cancer progression [2, 54]. The importance of melatonin in the regulation of several biological functions depends heavily on its lipophilic and hydrophilic traits that make it omnipresent in all cell compartments, principally in the nucleus [73]. Indeed, low levels of 6-sulfatoxymelatonin (6-SMT), the major metabolites of the hormone in urine [74], have been demonstrated to correlate with increased risk of breast cancer in postmenopausal women [75–77]. Furthermore, women with blindness or long sleep duration (elevated melatonin levels) present reduced breast cancer risk relative to normal women [78, 79].

Physiological blood concentration of melatonin blocked human leiomyosarcoma (soft tissue sarcoma) proliferation by inhibiting tumor metabolic and genetic pathways presumable by suppression of cellular cAMP levels *via* melatonin receptor [80]. In hepatocellular carcinoma-induced mice, melatonin treatment suppressed tumor cell proliferation through arresting the cell cycle [81]. The metastatic activity of oral squamous cell carcinoma was notably reduced by melatonin-mediated inhibition of tumor-associated neutrophils [82], inflammatory cells involved in promoting several solid tumors [83]. Similarly, the anti-oncogenic property of melatonin has been demonstrated also in other cancer types, including lung [84], gastric [85], ovarian [86], and colon [87], as well as breast cancers [88].

Melatonin could mediate its effects of cancer development *via* epigenetic modifications, particularly GDM [89]. Melatonin treatment to MCF-7 cell lines significantly increased DNA methylation that was associated with increased transcriptional levels of the tumor metastasis suppressor gene glypican-3 and decreased expression levels of the oncogenes EGR3 and POU4F2/Brn-3b [90]. In estrogen-receptor-related breast cancer, melatonin may decrease transcriptional levels of the aromatase gene (involved in the regulation of estrogen synthesis) by either methylation of the gene or deacetylation of the promoter gene [91]. Additionally, nocturnal melatonin treatment can rectify the induced DNA demethylation, tumor growth, and metastatic activity by both blue LED and fluorescent ALAN in 4T1 mammary cancer cell-inoculated female BALB/c mice [63, 64]. In a more recent study that evaluated the effects of ALAN and melatonin treatment at different spectral compositions in 4T1-inoculated BALB/c mice, a tissue-specific response in GDM was detected [19]. In this study, the tumor tissue manifested the most prominent changes in GDM showing an inverse wavelength-dependent correlation that was reversed by melatonin. Conversely, other tissues (e.g., lung, liver, and spleen) showed mixed results of positive, negative, or indifferent correlation between methylation levels and both wavelength and melatonin treatments [19]. Largely, melatonin may regulate epigenetic modifications in a number of tumor-related genes mainly by DNA methylation, but other modifications are also possible.

The strong association between ALAN, DNA hypo-methylation, and melatonin suppression may be of significant clinical importance. DNA methylation and melatonin can be utilized as biomarkers for detecting and preventing breast cancer development. The traditional diagnosis method for breast cancer is scanning by mammography, which is a useful technique to identify the growth of cancer. The mammography cannot predict risk for breast cancer as it indicates its existence, but trends in melatonin suppression and DNA methylation can provide a simple, noninvasive, and reliable tool for predicting cancer risk, particularly among a group of high-risk individuals for developing the disease such as night shift workers. Bearing in mind that epigenetic modifications are reversible [92], early treatment by melatonin or any other analogs [93] for individuals at high risk can be very effective in preventing breast cancer. We are aware today, that genetics factors such as breast cancer genes are not the major causes of the malignancy and other external factors are heavily involved. Therefore, much more attention should be given to environmental changes that link endocrinology with epigenetic modifications.

Collectively, in diurnal humans, circadian disruption enforced by activity impinging on the inactive period during the nighttime is recurrently associated with a number of health problems. However, a direct link between ALAN-induced circadian disruption and health risks is still difficult to clearly establish as most data are derived from epidemiological and nocturnal animal studies [94]. Therefore, integrating diurnal animal models of chronodisruption with epidemiological and nocturnal model studies would add a significant value in defining potential direct signal transduction pathways mediating the environmental exposure impacts on physiology and health. Consequently, we conducted a preliminary study to investigate the effects of hormonal manipulations in diurnal species on physiological and epigenetic regulations. This preliminary study is a first step in a large-scale study using diurnal mouse model to elucidate the association between ALAN-induced circadian disruption and the development of health problems at the behavioral, physiological, and molecular levels.

6. Physiological and epigenetic responses to melatonin and thyroxin in diurnal species

Bearing in mind that humans are diurnal, understanding the physiological and epigenetic response to ALAN in human disease can benefit significantly from using a diurnal species such as the fat sand rat (*Psammomys obesus*). This species is a good model because it is a photoperiodic species that responds to photoperiod with robust daily rhythms in a number of physiological functions, including body temperature, melatonin levels, and AA-NAT activity [95, 96]. Furthermore, *P. obesus* is a useful model for studying human health and diseases such as metabolic disorders, obesity, diabetes, inflammation, and cardiovascular impairment [97–100]. Since most previous studies on photoperiodic responses were conducted on nocturnal species, in our research center at the University of Haifa, we use *P. obesus* as a model for studying photoperiodic and hormonal manipulations. In *P. obesus*, melatonin and body temperature rhythms were diminished in response to constant dim blue light exposure, while melatonin treatment restored the disrupted rhythms [63]. Although the previous studies have clearly indicated that as a diurnal species, *P. obesus* can respond to photoperiod and light manipulations, the underling mechanism mediating the effect of the environmental changes remains unknown. An unanswered question is how melatonin and thyroxin interact to mediated environmental-induced epigenetic modifications. To answer this question, male *P. obesus* were acclimated to a long photoperiod cycle of 16L:8D at an ambient temperature of 24 ± 1°C and humidity of 45 ± 2%. Lights during the day were emitted from cool fluorescent lamps at 470 lux and 470 nm. Rats were caged individually and provided with ad libitum tap water and low energy diet. At the end of 3-week acclimation period, rats were either untreated, *i.p.* injected with melatonin, thyroxin, or melatonin and thyroxin in combination 3 h after the dark period onset (01:00 h). Hormones were daily administered for 3 weeks at a dose of 50 μg/kg for melatonin and 2 mg/kg for thyroxin. During the experimental period, body mass (W_b) was monitored every other day and urine samples were collected by a noninvasive method [19] at 4 h intervals over a 28 h period. Urine samples were used to measure the major metabolite of melatonin in urine, 6-SMT [101]. The urinary metabolite concentrations were assayed by enzyme-linked immunosorbent assay utilizing a commercial IBL kit (RE54031) following the manufacture's protocol. Finally, digit tips were collected from rats at the end of urine collection for DNA isolation (High pure PCR Template Preparation Kit, Roche) and subsequently for GDM analysis (MethylFlash™ Methylated DNA Quantificadion Kit, Epigentek). All experimental procedures were performed with the approval from the Ethics and Animal Care Committee of the University of Haifa.

The results showed that melatonin alone significantly increased W_b from day 1 compared with controls, but with a decreasing magnitude with time (**Figure 1A**). Mass gain on day 1 was approximately 1.5-fold higher compared with that at the last. T4 also increased W_b from day 1 to day 5 compared with controls, but with significantly lesser effect compared with melatonin. Thereafter, mass was decreased showing a moderate mass loss from day 13 to day 21 compared with controls. Thyroxin and melatonin in combination markedly decreased W_b with time compared with all other groups. Mass gain decreased from 0.46 ± 0.88% at day 1 to −20.21 ± 2.56% at day 21. Thyroxin can regulate W_b by increasing heat production through nonshivering thermogenesis by changing membrane permeability to sodium, increasing the pump activity to maintain cell homeostasis in brown adipose tissue, resulting in higher body temperature values and loss in W_b [102].

Melatonin may operate through increasing the amount of brown adipose tissue, thus increasing heat production by increasing energy expenditure. Melatonin and thyroxin in combination provoked considerably more mass loss than melatonin alone, suggesting that melatonin may act synergistically with thyroxin to evoke mass loss in rats, due to the combined effect of increasing energy expenditure.

Body temperature rhythms were notably altered only in response to T4 treatment, while melatonin alone and in combination with thyroxin had no effect on body temperature compared with controls (**Figure 1B**). Furthermore, the significant decrease in body temperature following treatments with thyroxin and melatonin in combination, compared with T4 alone, suggests that melatonin and thyroxin exert a significant antagonistic effect on body temperature.

Thyroxin treatment had no effect on mean 6-SMT levels but altered the daily rhythms with higher amplitude and delayed acrophase by approximately 2 h (**Figure 2A**). Finally, melatonin treatment elicited hypomethylation while thyroxin alone or thyroxin and melatonin in combination exerted comparable effects on GDM levels showing marked hypermethylation compared with control levels (**Figure 2B**). Similar to W_b, thyroxin and melatonin may have exerted synergistic effects on promoting DNA hypermethylation, but this effect did not reach statistical significance.

These results suggest that melatonin and thyroxin have a role in the regulation of body temperature and apparently metabolism, in which the former may attenuate metabolism and the latter may accelerate it. Both hormones exerted inverse effects on global DNA levels, suggesting that different transduction pathways are involved in the circadian regulation of body temperature in *P. obesus*. The results suggest also that change in body temperature is more sensitive to thyroxin treatment than melatonin, as the effect of the latter was masked in the combined treatment with the other hormone.

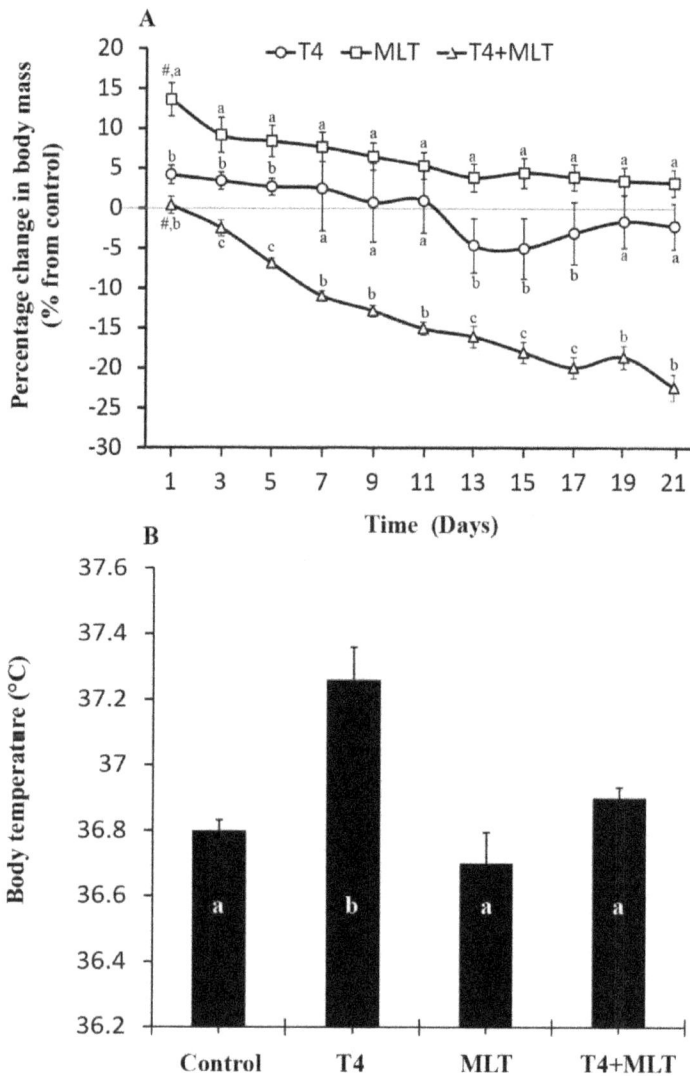

Figure 1.
Percentage change in body mass (A) and body temperature (B) in long-day acclimated P. obesus under four conditions: control no treatments, thyroxin (T4) treatment, melatonin (MLT) treatment, and combined treatment with T4 + MLT. Data are presented as mean ± standard error of nine animals. Different letters represent statistically significant difference among groups (Bonferroni, P < 0.01). # vs. day 21 (Bonferroni, P < 0.02).

However, in humans, melatonin may interact with the HPT axis to modulate the circadian rhythm of body temperature [104]. In mammals, the HPT axis plays a major role in several adaptive functions such as growth, development, metabolic rate, thermogenesis, heart rate, immune, and reproductive responses [105]. The HPT releasing and stimulating hormones as well as the thyroid hormones (T4 and T3) are under photoperiodic control presumably by the pars tuberalis of the adenohypophysis [106, 107]. In rats, T3 and T4 concentrations exhibit significant circadian rhythms with elevated levels during the dark period compared with the counterpart light period [108]. The nocturnal increase in the thyroid hormones was reported also in the rat pineal gland following an increase in type I 5′-iodothyronine deiodinase activity, which catalyzes the conversion of T4 to T3 [109]. Furthermore, the thyroid hormones are crucial photoperiodic regulators of several physiological

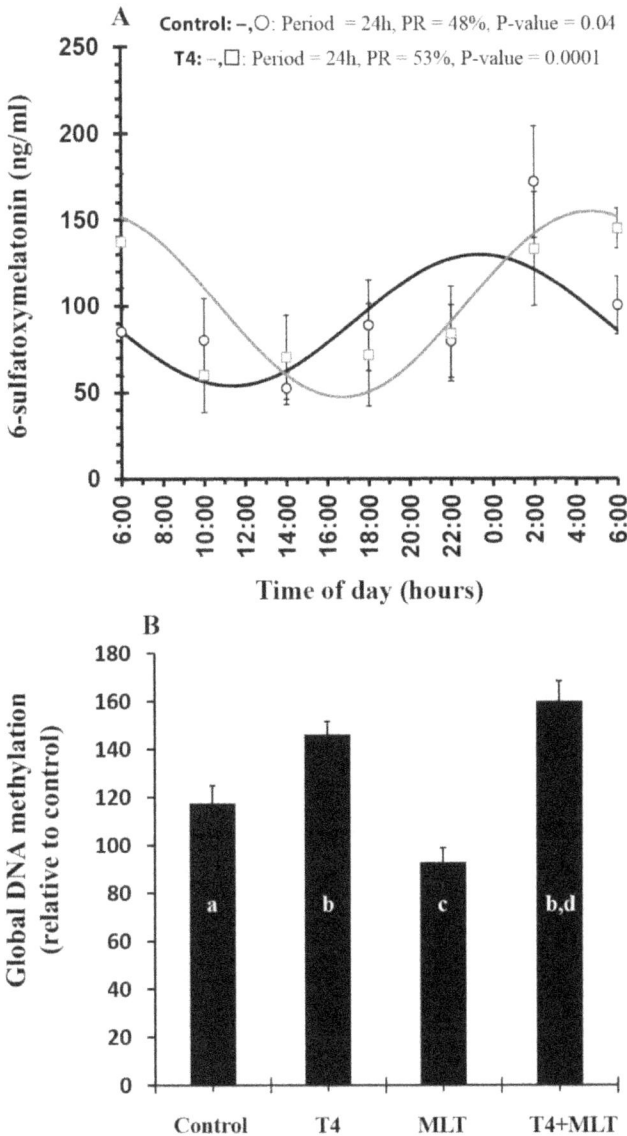

Figure 2.
Daily rhythms of urinary 6-sulfatoxymelatonin (A) and global DNA methylation (B) levels in long-day acclimated P. obesus under four conditions: control no treatments, thyroxin (T4) treatment, melatonin (MLT) treatment, and combined treatment with T4 + MLT. In panel A, the best-fitted cosine curve (black and gray lines) and Cosinor estimates (period, P-value, and percentage of the rhythm [PR]) are depicted [103]. The gray area in each plot represents the length of the dark period. Data are presented as mean ± standard error of seven to nine animals. Different letters represent statistically significant difference among groups (Bonferroni, P < 0.01).

processes including energy metabolism and reproduction [110, 111]. While the relation between the HPT axis and the photoperiodic system are well-characterized, there are limited studies on the effect of ALAN on the HPT axis. However, due to the link with the photoperiodic system, environmental perturbation of the circadian clock by ALAN is expected to alter the activity of the HPT axis, including the thyroid hormones. In hamsters under short-day photoperiod, low levels of ALAN elevated the levels of thyroid-stimulating-hormone (TSH) receptors causing advanced W_b and gonadal growth [112]. Continuous exposure to ALAN decreased

TSH, but increased both T3 and T4 in mice [113]. In birds, long-term exposure to ALAN increased both the blood levels of the thyroid hormones and W_b [114]. Overall, ALAN may induce aberrant epigenetic modifications by disrupting endocrine axes such as HPT axis that interacts with melatonin to manifest the adverse effects of the environmental exposure. However, the exact mechanism of action by which HPT axis may directly, or *via* melatonin, mediate the disruption effects of ALAN on the circadian system and promote downstream health risk is still unclear, and further efforts are warranted for elucidating it.

7. Conclusions

Currently, it is clear that electric light not only has remarkable anthropological advantages, but also severe adverse ecological and public health concerns. One of the most alerting impacts of ALAN on public health is the potential association between SWL exposure and cancer development, particularly in urbanized regions worldwide. ALAN effects are suggested to be mediated at the cellular level by inducing epigenetic modifications *via* nocturnal melatonin suppression. A schematic of ALAN-induced adverse effects is presented in **Figure 3**. Accordingly, light signals including ALAN are detected by ipRGCs and conveyed to the SCN by RHT. During a normal light dark cycle, melatonin is synthesized and secreted to the blood during the night, where it entrains central and peripheral oscillators to regulate normal physiological responses. Conversely, ALAN suppresses melatonin levels causing chronodisruption and misalignment in central and peripheral oscillators resulting in impaired physiological responses. The central and peripheral oscillators can be regulated directly by the melatonin signal or indirectly by modifying the body temperature rhythms [115]. In mice, daily variations in body temperature rhythms have been demonstrated to synchronize circadian gene expressions [116] and these central-controlled variations can be utilized to regulate variant peripheral circadian clocks in mammals [117]. Consequently, in diurnal species, thyroxin as an endocrine pathway is presumably involved in center circadian regulation of peripheral clocks by modifying body temperature daily rhythms.

These effects are presumably mediated by aberrant epigenetic modifications. Therefore, DNA methylations, which are a reversible modification in genes, triggered by melatonin, are a promising mechanism linking between environmental exposures like ALAN and hormonal/cellular pathway mediating carcinogenic activities like metastasis activity, tumor cell proliferation, and estrogen-related responses [89]. Melatonin may affect DNA methylation by modulating the activity of DNA methyltransferases involved in the regulation of gene expression by changing DNA methylation patterns. The well-established fact that different tissues present specific patterns of epigenetic modifications [118] may account for the observed tissue-specific effects of ALAN and melatonin on DNA methyl-transferase activity and GDM levels. Tissue differential effects on the activity of DNA methyl-transferases and GDM levels in response to ALAN exposure may present tissue-specific responses to genes that are involved in circadian regulation of several transduction pathways including cancer cell proliferation and metastatic activity. Since humans are diurnal species and most studies have been conducted on nocturnal animals, a diurnal experimental model should be of a great clinical interest. *P. obesus* may be very useful as a diurnal animal model for understanding the physiological and molecular effects of light pollution on public health. Melatonin suppression, GDM, and even thyroxin levels may present a significant clinical importance as a biomarker for early detection of cancer, particularly in individuals who are at increased risk of developing cancer by circadian disruption induced by excessive ALAN exposures. As epigenetic modifications are revisable, these biomarkers retain therapeutic value

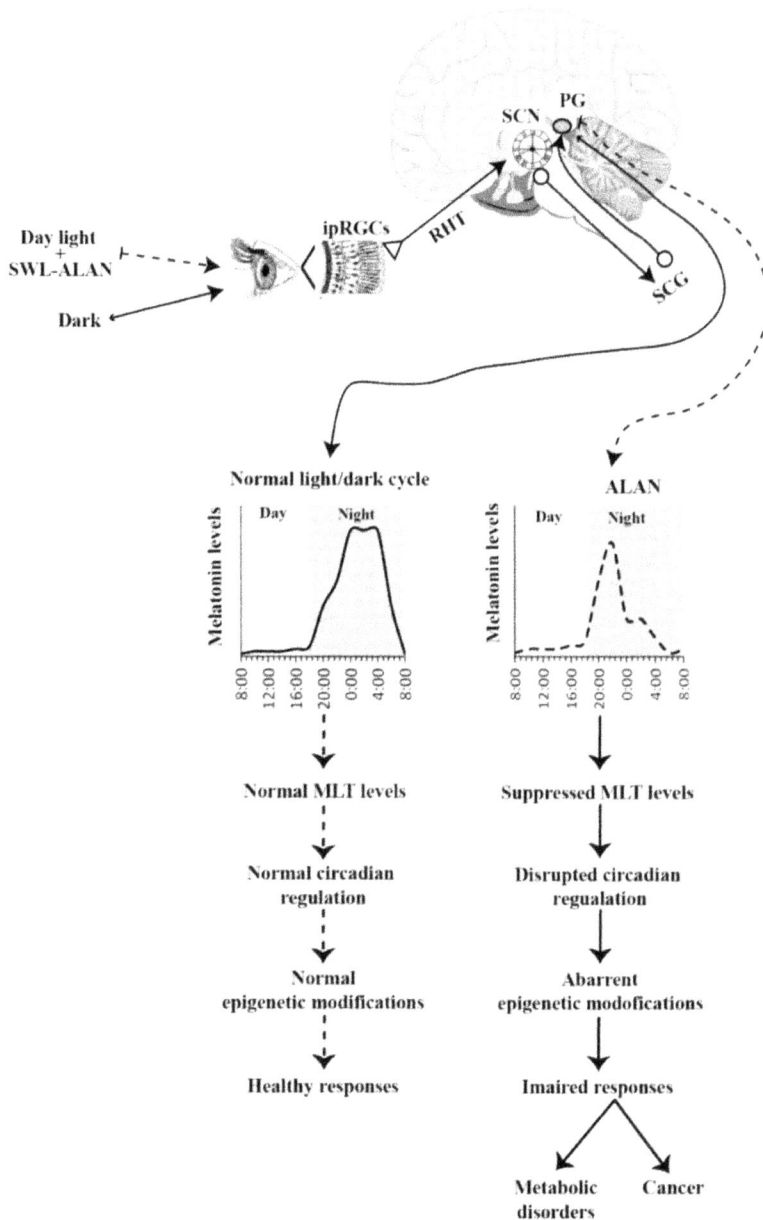

Figure 3.
Schematic representation of the mechanism of ALAN in eliciting adverse health effects. Light signal, including short wavelength ALAN (SWL-ALAN), is detected by intrinsically photosensitive retinal ganglion cells (ipRGCs) that propagate it to the SCN via the retinohypothalamic tract (RHT). Thereafter, the signal is transmitted to the pineal gland (PG) via superior cervical ganglion (SCG). Finally, melatonin is synthesized and secreted to circulation by the PG during the night, where it synchronizes peripheral clocks with the ambient photoperiod. Generally, ALAN suppresses nocturnal melatonin, in which adverse health impacts are generated by inducing aberrant epigenetic modifications.

for ALAN-induced cancer by gene demethylation. Finally, the accumulating data regarding the adverse effects of light pollution on ecology and heath compel us to take drastic and rapid measures to reduce light pollution by extreme regulation or at least reducing SWL emission by developing safe lightning technology.

Acknowledgements

The authors of this chapter would like to thank the Vice President and Dean of Research at the University of Haifa, Prof. Ido Izhaki for allocating the funding to the publication fee.

Dedication

This chapter is dedicated to the memory of Professor Abraham Haim, who passed away before publication of this work. His contribution was foremost among the authors of this chapter.

Abbreviations

ALAN	artificial light at night
AA-NAT	aryl-alkyl-amine-N-acetyltransferase
W_b	body mass
GDM	global DNA methylation
HIOMT	hydroxyindole-O-methyltransferase
SCN	hypothalamic suprachiasmatic nucleus
HPA	hypothalamic-pituitary-adrenal
HPG	hypothalamic-pituitary-gonadal
HPT	hypothalamic pituitary-thyroid axis
ipRGCs	intrinsically photosensitive retinal ganglion cells
LED	light-emitting diodes
RHT	retinohypothalamic tract
SWLs	short wavelengths
SCG	superior cervical ganglion
TSH	thyroid-stimulating hormone

Author details

Abraham Haim, Sinam Boynao and Abed Elsalam Zubidat*
The Israeli Center for Interdisciplinary Research in Chronobiology, University of Haifa, Haifa, Israel

*Address all correspondence to: zubidat3@013.net.il

IntechOpen

References

[1] Haim A, Portnov BA. LAN and breast cancer risk: Can we see a forest through the trees?—Response to "measurements of light at night (LAN) for a sample of female school teachers" by M. S. Rea, J. A. Brons, and M. G. Figueiro. Chronobiology International. 2011;**28**(8):734-736. DOI: 10.3109/07420528.2011.604591

[2] Zubidat AE, Haim A. Artificial light-at-night—A novel lifestyle risk factor for metabolic disorder and cancer morbidity. Journal of Basic and Clinical Physiology and Pharmacology. 2017;**28**(4):295-313. DOI: 10.1515/jbcpp-2016-0116

[3] Haim A, Scantlebury DM, Zubidat AE. The loss of ecosystem-services emerging from artificial light at night. Chronobiology International. 2018;**19**:1-3. DOI: 10.1080/07420528.2018.1534122

[4] Cinzano P, Falchi F, Elvidge CD. The first world atlas of the artificial night sky brightness. Monthly Notices of the Royal Astronomical Society. 2001;**328**(3):689-707. DOI: 10.1046/j.1365-8711.2001.04882.x

[5] Hölker F, Moss T, Griefahn B, Kloas W, Voigt CC, Henckel D, et al. The dark side of light: A transdisciplinary research agenda for light pollution policy. Ecology and Society. 2010;**15**:13. Available from: http://www.ecologyandsociety.org/vol15/iss4/art13/

[6] Navara KJ, Nelson RJ. The dark side of light at night: Physiological, epidemiological, and ecological consequences. Journal of Pineal Research. 2007;**43**(3):215-224

[7] Dominoni DM, Borniger JC, Nelson RJ. Light at night, clocks and health: From humans to wild organisms. Biological Letters. 2016;**12**(2):20160015. DOI: 10.1098/rsbl.2016.0015

[8] Russart KLG, Nelson RJ. Light at night as an environmental endocrine disruptor. Physiology and Behavior. 2018;**190**:82-89. DOI: 10.1016/j.physbeh.2017.08.029

[9] Owens ACS, Lewis SM. The impact of artificial light at night on nocturnal insects: A review and synthesis. Ecology and Evolution. 2018;**8**(22):11337-11358. DOI: 10.1002/ece3.4557

[10] Pulgar J, Zeballos D, Vargas J, Aldana M, Manriquez PH, Manriquez K, et al. Endogenous cycles, activity patterns and energy expenditure of an intertidal fish is modified by artificial light pollution at night (ALAN). Environmental Pollution. 2019;**244**:361-366. DOI: 10.1016/j.envpol.2018.10.063

[11] Gastón MS, Pereyra LC, Vaira M. Artificial light at night and captivity induces differential effects on leukocyte profile, body condition, and erythrocyte size of a diurnal toad. Journal of Experimental Zoology Part A: Ecological and Integrative Physiology. 2019;**331**(2):93-102. DOI: 10.1002/jez.2240

[12] Hu Z, Hu H, Huang Y. Association between nighttime artificial light pollution and sea turtle nest density along Florida coast: A geospatial study using VIIRS remote sensing data. Environmental Pollution. 2018;**239**:30-42. DOI: 10.1016/j.envpol.2018.04.021

[13] Dominoni DM, de Jong M, Bellingham M, O'Shaughnessy P, van Oers K, Robinson J, et al. Dose-response effects of light at night on the reproductive physiology of great tits (Parus major): Integrating morphological analyses with candidate gene expression. Journal of Experimental Zoology Part A: Ecological and Integrative Physiology. 2018;**329**(8-9):473-487. DOI: 10.1002/jez.2214

[14] Hoffmann J, Palme R, Eccard JA. Long-term dim light during nighttime changes activity patterns and space

use in experimental small mammal populations. Environmental Pollution. 2018l;**238**:844-851. DOI: 10.1016/j. envpol.2018.03.107

[15] Solano-Lamphar HA, Kocifaj M. Numerical research on the effects the skyglow could have in phytochromes and RQE photoreceptors of plants. Journal of Environmental Management. 2018;**209**:484-494. DOI: 10.1016/j. jenvman.2017.12.036

[16] Nelson RJ, Chbeir S. Dark matters: Effects of light at night on metabolism. Proceedings of the Nutrition Society. 2018;**77**(30):223-229. DOI: 10.1017/S0029665118000198

[17] Abay KA, Amare M. Night light intensity and women's body weight: Evidence from Nigeria. Economics and Human Biology. 2018;**31**:238-248. DOI: 10.1016/j.ehb.2018.09.001

[18] Garcia-Saenz A, Sánchez de Miguel A, Espinosa A, Valentin A, Aragonés N, Llorca J, et al. Evaluating the association between artificial light-at-night exposure and breast and prostate cancer risk in Spain (MCC-Spain Study). Environmental Health Perspectives. 2018;**126**:047011. DOI: 10.1289/EHP1837

[19] Zubidat AE, Fares B, Fares F, Haim A. Artificial light at night of different spectral compositions differentially affects tumor growth in mice: Interaction with melatonin and epigenetic pathways. Cancer Control. 2018;**25**(1):1073274818812908. DOI: 10.1177/1073274818812908

[20] Haim A, Heth G, Pratt H, Nevo E. Photoperiodic effects on thermoregulation in a 'blind' subterranean mammal. Journal Experimental Biology. 1983;**107**:59-64

[21] Zubidat AE, Nelson RJ, Haim A. Spectral and duration sensitivity to light-at-night in 'blind' and sighted rodent species. Journal of Experimental Biology. 2011;**214**(Pt 19):3206-3217. DOI: 10.1242/jeb.058883

[22] Matynia A. Blurring the boundaries of vision: Novel functions of intrinsically photosensitive retinal ganglion cells. Journal of Experimental Neuroscience. 2013;**7**:43-50. DOI: 10.4137/JEN.S11267

[23] Collin SP, Davies WL, Hart NS, Hunt DM. The evolution of early vertebrate photoreceptors. Philosophical Transactions of The Royal Society B Biological Sciences. 2009;**364**(1531):2925-2940. DOI: 10.1098/rstb.2009.0099

[24] Detwiler PB. Phototransduction in retinal ganglion cells. Yale Journal of Biology and Medicine. 2018;**91**(1):49-52

[25] Hannibal J, Christiansen AT, Heegaard S, Fahrenkrug J, Kiilgaard JF. Melanopsin expressing human retinal ganglion cells: Subtypes, distribution, and intraretinal connectivity. Journal of Comparative Neurology. 2017;**525**(8):1934-1961. DOI: 10.1002/cne.24181

[26] Moore RY. Neural control of the pineal gland. Behavioural Brain Research. 1996;**73**(1-2):125-130

[27] Perreau-Lenz S, Kalsbeek A, Van Der Vliet J, Pévet P, Buijs RM. In vivo evidence for a controlled offset of melatonin synthesis at dawn by the suprachiasmatic nucleus in the rat. Neuroscience. 2005;**130**(3):797-803

[28] Klein DC. Arylalkylamine N-acetyltransferase: "the Timezyme". Journal of Biological Chemistry. 2007;**282**(7):4233-4237

[29] Klein DC, Coon SL, Roseboom PH, Weller JL, Bernard M, Gastel JA, et al. The melatonin rhythm-generating enzyme: Molecular regulation of

serotonin N-acetyltransferase in the pineal gland. Recent Progress in Hormone Research. 1997;**52**:307-357

[30] Maronde E, Stehle JH. The mammalian pineal gland: Known facts, unknown facets. Trends in Endocrinology and Metabolism. 2007;**18**(11):142-149

[31] Ribelayga C, Garidou ML, Malan A, Gauer F, Calgari C, Pévet P, et al. Photoperiodic control of the rat pineal arylalkylamine-N-acetyltransferase and hydroxyindole-O-methyltransferase gene expression and its effect on melatonin synthesis. Journal of Biological Rhythms. 1999;**14**(2):105-115

[32] Thapan K, Arendt J, Skene DJ. An action spectrum for melatonin suppression: Evidence for a novel non-rod, non-cone photoreceptor system in humans. Journal of Physiology. 2001;**535**(Pt 1):261-267

[33] Cajochen C, Münch M, Kobialka S, Kräuchi K, Steiner R, Oelhafen P, et al. High sensitivity of human melatonin, alertness, thermoregulation, and heart rate to short wavelength light. Journal of Clinical Endocrinology and Metabolism. 2005;**90**(3):1311-1316

[34] Brainard GC, Lewy AJ, Menaker M, Fredrickson RH, Miller LS, Weleber RG, et al. Dose-response relationship between light irradiance and the suppression of plasma melatonin in human volunteers. Brain Research. 1988;**454**(1-2):212-218

[35] Falchi F, Cinzano P, Elvidge CD, Keith DM, Haim A. Limiting the impact of light pollution on human health, environment and stellar visibility. Journal of Environmental Management. 2011;**92**(10):2714-2722. DOI: 10.1016/j.jenvman.2011.06.029

[36] Aubé M, Roby J, Kocifaj M. Evaluating potential spectral impacts of various artificial lights on melatonin suppression, photosynthesis, and star visibility. PLoS One. 2013;**8**:e67798. DOI: 10.1371/journal.pone.0067798

[37] West KE, Jablonski MR, Warfield B, Cecil KS, James M, Ayers MA, et al. Blue light from light-emitting diodes elicits a dose-dependent suppression of melatonin in humans. Journal of Applied Physiology. 2011;**110**(3):619-626. DOI: 10.1152/japplphysiol.01413.2009

[38] Walsh CM, Prendergast RL, Sheridan JT, Murphy BA. Blue light from light-emitting diodes directed at a single eye elicits a dose-dependent suppression of melatonin in horses. The Veterinary Journal. 2013;**196**(2):231-235. DOI: 10.1016/j.tvjl.2012.09.003

[39] Figueiro MG, Bierman A, Rea MS. A train of blue light pulses delivered through closed eyelids suppresses melatonin and phase shifts the human circadian system. Nature and Science of Sleep. 2013;**5**:133-141. DOI: 10.2147/NSS.S52203

[40] Figueiro MG, Plitnick B, Rea MS. Pulsing blue light through closed eyelids: Effects on acute melatonin suppression and phase shifting of dim light melatonin onset. Nature and Science of Sleep. 2014;**6**:149-156. DOI: 10.2147/NSS.S73856

[41] Haim A, Portnov BA. Light Pollution as a New Risk Factor for Human Breast and Prostate Cancers. Dordecht: Springer Science + Buisness Media; 2013. DOI: 10.1007/978-94-007-6220-6_1

[42] Ando K, Kripke DF. Light attenuation by the human eyelid. Biological Psychiatry. 1996;**39**(1):22-25

[43] Bierman A, Figueiro MG, Rea MS. Measuring and predicting eyelid spectral transmittance. Journal of Biomedical Optics. 2011;**16**:067011. DOI: 10.1117/1.3593151

[44] Figueiro MG, Wood B, Plitnick B, Rea MS. The impact of light from computer monitors on melatonin levels in college students. Neuro Endocrinology Letters. 2011;**32**(2):158-163

[45] Wood B, Rea MS, Plitnick B, Figueiro MG. Light level and duration of exposure determine the impact of self-luminous tablets on melatonin suppression. Applied Ergonomics. 2013;**44**(2):237-240. DOI: 10.1016/j.apergo.2012.07.008

[46] Green A, Cohen-Zion M, Haim A, Dagan Y. Evening light exposure to computer screens disrupts human sleep, biological rhythms, and attention abilities. Chronobiology International. 2017;**34**(7):855-865. DOI: 10.1080/07420528.2017.1324878

[47] Gaston KJ, Duffy JP, Gaston S, Bennie J, Davies TW. Human alteration of natural light cycles: Causes and ecological consequences. Oecologia. 2014;**76**(4):917-931. DOI: 10.1007/s00442-014-3088-2

[48] Kyba CCM, Kuester T, Sánchez de Miguel A, Baugh K, Jechow A, Hölker F, et al. Artificially lit surface of Earth at night increasing in radiance and extent. Science Advances. 2017;**3**:e1701528. DOI: 10.1126/sciadv.1701528

[49] AMA. Human and environment effects of light emitting diode (LED). Community Lighting. 2016. Available from: https://circadianlight.com/images/pdfs/newscience/American-Medical-Association-2016-Health-Effects-of-LED-Street-Lighting [Accessed: 28 December 2019]

[50] Wingfield JC. Environmental endocrinology: Insights into the diversity of regulatory mechanisms in life cycles. Integrative and Comparative Biology. 2018;**58**(4):790-799. DOI: 10.1093/icb/icy081

[51] Ouyang JQ, Davies S, Dominoni D. Hormonally mediated effects of artificial light at night on behavior and fitness: linking endocrine mechanisms with function. Journal of Experimental Biology. 2018;**221**(Pt 6):1-11. pii: jeb156893. DOI: 10.1242/jeb.156893

[52] Zhang X, Ho SM. Epigenetics meets endocrinology. Journal of Molecular Endocrinology. 2011;**46**(1):R11-R32

[53] Fleisch AF, Wright RO, Baccarelli AA. Environmental epigenetics: A role in endocrine disease? Journal of Molecular Endocrinology. 2012;**49**(2):R61-R67. DOI: 10.1530/JME-12-0066

[54] Touitou Y, Reinberg A, Touitou D. Association between light at night, melatonin secretion, sleep deprivation, and the internal clock: Health impacts and mechanisms of circadian disruption. Life Science. 2017;**173**: 94-106. DOI: 10.1016/j.lfs.2017.02.008

[55] Kloog I, Haim A, Stevens RG, Portnov BA. Global co-distribution of light at night (LAN) and cancers of prostate, colon, and lung in men. Chronobiology International. 2009;**26**(1):108-125. DOI: 10.1080/07420520802694020

[56] Kloog I, Stevens RG, Haim A, Portnov BA. Nighttime light level co-distributes with breast cancer incidence worldwide. Cancer Causes & Control. 2010;**21**(12):2059-2068. DOI: 10.1007/s10552-010-9624-4

[57] Kim YJ, Park MS, Lee E, Choi JW. High incidence of breast cancer in light-polluted areas with spatial effects in Korea. Asian Pacific Journal of Cancer Prevention. 2016;**17**(1):361-367

[58] Keshet-Sitton A, Or-Chen K, Yitzhak S, Tzabary I, Haim A. Light and the City: Breast cancer risk factors differ between urban and rural women in Israel. Integrative Cancer Therapies.

2017;**16**(2):176-187. DOI: 10.1177/1534735416660194

[59] Anderson LE, Morris JE, Sasser LB, Stevens RG. Effect of constant light on DMBA mammary tumorigenesis in rats. Cancer Letters. 2000;**148**(2):121-126

[60] Blask DE, Dauchy RT, Sauer LA, Krause JA, Brainard GC. Growth and fatty acid metabolism of human breast cancer (MCF-7) xenografts in nude rats: Impact of constant light-induced nocturnal melatonin suppression. Breast Cancer Research and Treatment. 2003;**79**(3):313-320

[61] Cos S, Mediavilla D, Martínez-Campa C, González A, Alonso-González C, Sánchez-Barceló EJ. Exposure to light-at-night increases the growth of DMBA-induced mammary adenocarcinomas in rats. Cancer Letters. 2006;**235**(2):266-271

[62] Vinogradova IA, Anisimov VN, Bukalev AV, Ilyukha VA, Khizhkin EA, Lotosh TA, et al. Circadian disruption induced by light-at-night accelerates aging and promotes tumorigenesis in young but not in old rats. Aging (Albany NY). 2010;**2**(2):82-92

[63] Schwimmer H, Metzer A, Pilosof Y, Szyf M, Machnes ZM, Fares F, et al. Light at night and melatonin have opposite effects on breast cancer tumors in mice assessed by growth rates and global DNA methylation. Chronobiology International. 2014;**31**(1):144-150. DOI: 10.3109/07420528.2013.842925

[64] Zubidat AE, Fares B, Faras F, Haim A. Melatonin functioning through DNA methylation to constrict breast cancer growth accelerated by blue LED light at night in 4T1 tumor bearing mice. Journal of Cancer Biology and Therapeutics. 2015;**1**(2):57-73. DOI: 10.18314/gjct.v1i2.35

[65] Karsli-Ceppioglu S, Dagdemir A, Judes G, Ngollo M, Penault-Llorca F, Pajon A,

et al. Epigenetic mechanisms of breast cancer: An update of the current knowledge. Epigenomics. 2014;**6**(6):651-664. DOI: 10.2217/epi.14.59

[66] Xiang TX, Yuan Y, Li LL, Wang ZH, Dan LY, Chen Y, et al. Aberrant promoter CpG methylation and its translational applications in breast cancer. Chinse Journal Cancer. 2013;**32**(10):12-20. DOI: 10.5732/cjc.011.10344

[67] Ross JP, Rand KN, Molloy PL. Hypomethylation of repeated DNA sequences in cancer. Epigenomics. 2010;**2**(2):245-269. DOI: 10.2217/epi.10.2

[68] Ogishima T, Shiina H, Breault JE, Tabatabai L, Bassett WW, Enokida H, et al. Increased heparanase expression is caused by promoter hypomethylation and up-regulation of transcriptional factor early growth response-1 in human prostate cancer. Clinical Cancer Research. 2005;**11**(3):1028-1036

[69] Loriot A, Van Tongelen A, Blanco J, Klaessens S, Cannuyer J, van Baren N, et al. A novel cancer-germline transcript carrying pro-metastatic miR-105 and TET-targeting miR-767 induced by DNA hypomethylation in tumors. Epigenetics. 2014;**9**(8):1163-1171. DOI: 10.4161/epi.29628

[70] Soares J, Pinto AE, Cunha CV, André S, Barão I, Sousa JM, et al. Global DNA hypomethylation in breast carcinoma: Correlation with prognostic factors and tumor progression. Cancer. 1999;**85**(1):112-118

[71] Jackson K, Yu MC, Arakawa K, Fiala E, Youn B, Fiegl H, et al. DNA hypomethylation is prevalent even in low-grade breast cancers. Cancer Biology and Therapy. 2004;**3**(12):1225-1231

[72] Stevens RG. Electric power use and breast cancer: A hypothesis.

American Journal of Epidemiology.
1987;**125**(4):556-561

[73] Reiter RJ. Functional pleiotropy
of the neurohormone melatonin:
Antioxidant protection and
neuroendocrine regulation.
Frontiers in Neuroendocrinology.
1995;**16**(4):383-415

[74] Middleton B. Measurement of
melatonin and 6-sulphatoxymelatonin.
Methods in Molecular Biology.
2013;**1065**:171-199. DOI:
10.1007/978-1-62703-616-0_11

[75] Schernhammer ES, Hankinson SE.
Urinary melatonin levels and
postmenopausal breast cancer risk
in the Nurses' Health Study cohort.
Cancer Epidemiology, Biomarkers and
Prevention. 2009;**18**(1):74-79.
DOI: 10.1158/1055-9965.EPI-08-0637

[76] Basler M, Jetter A, Fink D, Seifert B,
Kullak-Ublick GA, Trojan A. Urinary
excretion of melatonin and association
with breast cancer: Meta-analysis and
review of the literature. Breast Care
(Basel). 2014;**9**(3):182-187.
DOI: 10.1159/000363426

[77] Brown SB, Hankinson SE, Eliassen AH,
Reeves KW, Qian J, Arcaro KF, et al.
Urinary melatonin concentration and
the risk of breast cancer in Nurses'
Health Study II. American Journal
Epidemiology. 2015;**181**(3):155-162.
DOI: 10.1093/aje/kwu261

[78] Kliukiene J, Tynes T, Andersen A.
Risk of breast cancer among Norwegian
women with visual impairment. British
Journal of Cancer. 2001;**84**(3):
397-399

[79] Wu AH, Wang R, Koh WP,
Stanczyk FZ, Lee HP, Yu MC. Sleep
duration, melatonin and breast cancer
among Chinese women in Singapore.
Carcinogenesis. 2008;**29**(6):
1244-1248. DOI: 10.1093/carcin/bgn100

[80] Mao L, Dauchy RT, Blask DE,
Dauchy EM, Slakey LM, Brimer S,
et al. Melatonin suppression of aerobic
glycolysis (Warburg effect), survival
signalling and metastasis in human
leiomyosarcoma. Journal Pineal
Research. 2016;**60**(2):167-177. DOI:
10.1111/jpi.12298

[81] Sánchez DI, González-Fernández B,
Crespo I, San-Miguel B, Álvarez M,
González-Gallego J, et al. Melatonin
modulates dysregulated circadian
clocks in mice with diethylnitrosamine-
induced hepatocellular carcinoma. Jornal
of Pineal Research. 2018;**65**(3):e12506.
DOI: 10.1111/jpi.12506

[82] Lu H, Wu B, Ma G, Zheng D, Song R,
Huang E, Mao M, Lu B. Melatonin
represses oral squamous cell carcinoma
metastasis by inhibiting tumor-
associated neutrophils. American
Journal of Translational Research.
2017;**9**:5361-5374

[83] Hurt B, Schulick R, Edil B, El Kasmi KC,
Barnett C Jr. Cancer-promoting
mechanisms of tumor-associated
neutrophils. The American Journal of
Surgery. 2017;**214**(5):938-944.
DOI: 10.1016/j.amjsurg.2017.08.003

[84] Fan C, Pan Y, Yang Y, Di S, Jiang
S, Ma Z, et al. HDAC1 inhibition by
melatonin leads to suppression of lung
adenocarcinoma cells via induction
of oxidative stress and activation of
apoptotic pathways. Journal of Pineal
Research. 2015;**59**(3):321-333. DOI:
10.1111/jpi.12261

[85] Li W, Fan M, Chen Y, Zhao Q, Song C,
Yan Y, et al. Melatonin induces cell
apoptosis in AGS cells through the
activation of JNK and P38 MAPK
and the suppression of nuclear
factor-kappa B: A novel therapeutic
implication for gastric cancer.
Cellular Physiology and Biochemistry.
2015;**37**(6):2323-2338.
DOI: 10.1159/000438587

[86] Akbarzadeh M, Movassaghpour AA, Ghanbari H, Kheirandish M, Fathi Maroufi N, Rahbarghazi R, et al. The potential therapeutic effect of melatonin on human ovarian cancer by inhibition of invasion and migration of cancer stem cells. Scientific Reports. 2017;7:17062. DOI: 10.1038/s41598-017-16940-y

[87] Bakalova R, Zhelev Z, Shibata S, Nikolova B, Aoki I, Higashi T. Impressive suppression of colon cancer growth by triple combination SN38/EF24/melatonin: "oncogenic" versus "onco-suppressive" reactive oxygen species. Anticancer Research. 2017;37(10):5449-5458

[88] Mao L, Summers W, Xiang S, Yuan L, Dauchy RT, Reynolds A, et al. Melatonin represses metastasis in Her2-postive human breast cancer cells by suppressing RSK2 expression. Molecular Cancer Research. 2016;14(11):1159-1169

[89] Haim A, Zubidat AE. Artificial light at night: Melatonin as a mediator between the environment and epigenome. Philosophical transactions of the Royal Society of London. Series B, Biological sciences. 2015;370(1667): 1-7. pii: 20140121. DOI: 10.1098/rstb.2014.0121

[90] Lee SE, Kim SJ, Yoon HJ, Yu SY, Yang H, Jeong SI, et al. Genome-wide profiling in melatonin-exposed human breast cancer cell lines identifies differentially methylated genes involved in the anticancer effect of melatonin. Journal of Pineal Research. 2013;54(1):80-88. DOI: 10.1111/j.1600-079X.2012.01027.x

[91] Korkmaz A, Sanchez-Barcelo EJ, Tan DX, Reiter RJ. Role of melatonin in the epigenetic regulation of breast cancer. Breast Cancer Research and Treatment. 2009;115(1):13-27. DOI: 10.1007/s10549-008-0103-5

[92] Bennett RL, Licht JD. Targeting epigenetics in cancer. Annual Review of Pharmacology and Toxicology. 2018;58:187-207. DOI: 10.1146/annurev-pharmtox-010716-105106

[93] Gatti G, Lucini V, Dugnani S, Calastretti A, Spadoni G, Bedini A, Rivara S, Mor M, Canti G, Scaglione F, Bevilacqua A. Antiproliferative and pro-apoptotic activity of melatonin analogues on melanoma and breast cancer cells. Oncotarget. 2017; 8:68338-68353. DOI: 10.18632/oncotarget.20124.

[94] Nunez AA, Yan L, Smale L. The cost of activity during the rest phase: Animal models and theoretical perspectives. Frontiers in Endocrinology (Lausanne). 2018;9:72. DOI: 10.3389/fendo.2018.00072

[95] Neuman A, Gothilf Y, Haim A, Ben-Aharon G, Zisapel N. Nocturnal patterns and up-regulated excretion of the melatonin metabolite 6-sulfatoxymelatonin in the diurnal rodent *Psammomys obesus* post-weaning under a short photoperiod. Comparative Biochemistry and Physiology Part A: Molecular & Integrative Physiology. 2005;142(3):297-307

[96] Schwimmer H, Mursu N, Haim A. Effects of light and melatonin treatment on body temperature and melatonin secretion daily rhythms in a diurnal rodent, the fat sand rat. Chronobiology International. 2010;27(7):1401-1419. DOI: 10.3109/07420528.2010.505355

[97] Bouderba S, Sanchez-Martin C, Villanueva GR, Detaille D, Koceïr EA. Beneficial effects of silibinin against the progression of metabolic syndrome, increased oxidative stress, and liver steatosis in *Psammomys obesus*, a relevant animal model of human obesity and diabetes. Journal of Diabetes. 2014;6(2):184-192. DOI: 10.1111/1753-0407.12083

[98] Sihali-Beloui O, El-Aoufi S, Maouche B, Marco S. *Psammomys obesus*,

a uniquemodel of metabolic syndrome, inflammation and autophagy in the pathologic development of hepatic steatosis. Comptes Rendus Biologies. 2016;**339**(11-12):475-486. DOI: 10.1016/j.crvi.2016.08.001

[99] Gouaref I, Detaille D, Wiernsperger N, Khan NA, Leverve X, Koceir EA. The desert gerbil *Psammomys obesus* as a model for metformin-sensitive nutritional type 2 diabetes to protect hepatocellular metabolic damage: Impact of mitochondrial redox state. PLoS One. 2017;**12**:e0172053. DOI: 10.1371/journal.pone.0172053

[100] Chaudhary R, Walder KR, Hagemeyer CE, Kanwar JR. *Psammomys obesus*: A atural diet-controlled model for diabetes and cardiovascular diseases. Current Atherosclerosis Reports. 2018;**20**(9):46. DOI: 10.1007/s11883-018-0746-6

[101] de Almeida EA, Di Mascio P, Harumi T, Spence DW, Moscovitch A, Hardeland R, et al. Measurement of melatonin in body fluids: Standards, protocols and procedures. Child's Nervous System. 2011;**27**(6):879-891. DOI: 10.1007/s00381-010-1278-8

[102] Bianco AC, McAninch EA. The role of thyroid hormone and brown adipose tissue in energy homoeostasis. Lancet Diabetes and Endocrinology. 2013;**1**(3):250-258. DOI: 10.1016/S2213-8587(13)70069-X

[103] Nelson W, Tong Y, Lee J, Halberg F. Methods for cosinor-rhythmometry. Chronobiologia. 1979;**6**(4):305-323

[104] Mazzoccoli G, Giuliani A, Carughi S, De Cata A, Puzzolante F, La Viola M, et al. The hypothalamic-pituitary-thyroid axis and melatonin in humans: Possible interactions in the control of body temperature. Neuro Endocrinology Letters. 2004;**25**(5):368-372

[105] Zoeller RT, Tan SW, Tyl RW. General background on the hypothalamic-pituitary-thyroid (HPT) axis. Critical Reviews in Toxicology. 2007;**37**(1-2):11-53

[106] Dardente H, Hazlerigg DG, Ebling FJ. Thyroid hormone and seasonal rhythmicity. Frontiers Endocrinology (Lausanne). 2014;**5**:19. DOI: 10.3389/fendo.2014.00019

[107] Korf HW. Signaling pathways to and from the hypophysial pars tuberalis, an important center for the control of seasonal rhythms. General and Comparative Endocrinology. 2018;**258**:236-243. DOI: 10.1016/j.ygcen.2017.05.011

[108] Campos-Barros A, Musa A, Flechner A, Hessenius C, Gaio U, Meinhold H, et al. Evidence for circadian variations of thyroid hormone concentrations and type II 5′-iodothyronine deiodinase activity in the rat central nervous system. Journal of Neurochemistry. 1997;**68**(2):795-803

[109] Soutto M, Guerrero JM, Osuna C, Molinero P. Nocturnal increases in the triiodothyronine/thyroxine ratio in the rat thymus and pineal gland follow increases of type II 5′-deiodinase activity. The International Journal of Biochemistry and Cell Biology. 1998;**30**(2):235-241

[110] Hut RA. Photoperiodism: Shall EYA compare thee to a summer's day? Current Biology. 2011;**21**(1):R22-R25. DOI: 10.1016/j.cub.2010.11.060

[111] Wood S, Loudon A. Clocks for all seasons: Unwinding the roles and mechanisms of circadian and interval timers in the hypothalamus and pituitary. Journal of Endocrinology. 2014;**222**(2):R39-R59. DOI: 10.1530/JOE-14-0141

[112] Ikeno T, Weil ZM, Nelson RJ. Dim light at night disrupts the short-day

response in Siberian hamsters. General and Comparative Endocrinology. 2014;**197**:56-64. DOI: 10.1016/j. ygcen.2013.12.005

[113] Maroni MJ, Capri KM, Cushman AV, Monteiro De Pina IK, Chasse MH, Seggio JA. Constant light alters serum hormone levels related to thyroid function in male CD-1 mice. Chronobiology International. 2018;**35**(10):1456-1463. DOI: 10.1080/07420528.2018

[114] Yang Y, Yu Y, Yang B, Zhou H, Pan J. Physiological responses to daily light exposure. Scientific Reports. 2016;**6**:24808. DOI: 10.1038/srep24808

[115] Borniger JC, Maurya SK, Periasamy M, Nelson RJ. Acute dim light at night increases body mass, alters metabolism, and shifts core body temperature circadian rhythms. Chronobiology International. 2014;**31**(8):917-925. DOI: 10.3109/07420528.2014.926911

[116] Saini C, Morf J, Stratmann M, Gos P, Schibler U. Simulated body temperature rhythms reveal the phase-shifting behavior and plasticity of mammalian circadian oscillators. Genes and Development. 2012;**26**(6):567-580. DOI: 10.1101/ gad.183251.111

[117] Brown SA, Zumbrunn G, Fleury-Olela F, Preitner N, Schibler U. Rhythms of mammalian body temperature can sustain peripheral circadian clocks. Current Biology. 2002;**12**(18): 1574-1583. Available from: https:// linkinghub.elsevier.com/retrieve/pii/ S0960-9822(02)01145-4

[118] Zhang M, Xu C, von Wettstein D, Liu B. Tissue-specific differences in cytosine methylation and their association with differential gene expression in sorghum. Plant Physiology. 2011;**156**(4):1955-1966. DOI: 10.1104/pp.111.176842

A Hypothesis to Explain How the DNA of Elderly People Is Prone to Damage: Genome-Wide Hypomethylation Drives Genomic Instability in the Elderly by Reducing Youth-Associated Gnome-Stabilizing DNA Gaps

Apiwat Mutirangura

Abstract

Epigenetic changes are how the DNA of elderly people is prone to damage. One role of DNA methylation is to prevent DNA damage. In the elderly and those with aging-associated noncommunicable diseases (NCDs), DNA shows reduced methylation; consequently, the aging genome is unstable and accumulates DNA damage. While the DNA damage response (DDR) of the direct intracellular machinery repairs DNA lesions, too much DDR halts cell proliferation, and promotes senescence. Therefore, genome-wide hypomethylation drives genomic instability, causing aging-associated disease phenotypes. However, the mechanism is unknown. Independent of DNA replication, the eukaryotic genome retains a certain amount of endogenous DNA double-strand breaks (EDSBs), called physiologic replication-independent EDSBs (Phy-RIND-EDSBs), that possess physiologic function. Phy-RIND-EDSBs are reduced in aging yeast, and low levels of Phy-RIND-EDSBs decrease cell viability and increase DNA damage. Thus, Phy-RIND-EDSBs have a biological role as youth-associated genomic-stabilizing DNA gaps. In humans, Phy-RIND-EDSBs are located in the hypermethylated genome. Because the genomes of aging people are hypomethylated, the elderly should also have a low level of Phy-RIND-EDSBs. Based on this evidence, I hypothesize that in the human Phy-RIND-EDSBs, reduction is a molecular process that mediates the genome-wide hypomethylation driving genomic instability, which is a nidus pathogenesis mechanism of human body deterioration in aging-associated NCDs.

Keywords: genome-wide hypomethylation, genomic instability, global hypomethylation, DNA damage, youth-associated genomic-stabilizing DNA gaps, youth-DNA-GAPs, physiological replication-independent endogenous DNA double-strand breaks, RIND-EDSBs, Phy-RIND-EDSBs, aging

1. Introduction

As people age, their bodies begin to deteriorate. Understanding how changes in the DNA of aging people affect cellular function will be an important clue for future prevention and treatment of age-associated noncommunicable diseases (NCDs). Genomic instability, a hallmark of cancer and aging, is defined as a high frequency of mutations within the genome [1, 2]. In cancer, the permanent alteration of the nucleotide sequence of DNA, or mutations, occurring in proto-oncogenes and tumor suppressor genes lead to cancer development and progression. In the aging process, however, the accumulation of DNA damage, which is an abnormal chemical structure in DNA and includes base modification, base loss, and DNA breaks (which are precursors of mutations), stimulates the DNA damage repair signal (DDR) to induce cells to repair DNA damage [3, 4]. Nevertheless, DDR arrests the cell cycle, rewires cellular metabolism, promotes senescence, and initiates programmed cell death. As a result, too much DDR drives the cellular aging process [3, 4]. Accumulation of DNA damage is found in the elderly and people with age-associated NCDs (**Figure 1**) [5]. Therefore, DNA damage accumulation is a crucial molecular pathogenic mechanism of the aging process. However, the mechanism by which DNA damage spontaneously accumulates in the aging genome remains to be explored.

Both epigenetic marks and DNA damage or lesions are temporary modifications of DNA. However, both are produced by different mechanisms and play roles in genomic instability in opposite directions. Epigenetic marks are produced by biological processes and possess physiological functions [6, 7]. For example, DNA methylation or methyl CpG is produced by DNA methyltransferase. The molecular function of methyl CpG is to interact with a protein such as methyl-CpG-binding protein. This interaction forms a cascade of molecular biological processes for gene regulation control and genomic stability. DNA lesions, on the other hand, are produced by endogenous or exogenous hazards [8]. For example, pyrimidine dimers, one type of DNA lesion, are formed via photochemical reactions such as exposure to UV light. DNA damage is converted into a mutation during subsequent replication, so accumulation of DNA damage leads to genomic instability. This chapter describes that genomic instability in the elderly should occur by the alteration of epigenetic marks leading to spontaneous accumulation of DNA damage.

Global DNA hypomethylation is an epigenetic change in the elderly and people with NCDs that promotes genomic instability [9–13]. However, the underlying mechanism of how the hypomethylated genome accumulates DNA damage is unknown [14]. In 2008, my group discovered an unprecedented type of endogenous DNA double-strand break (EDSB). These breaks are found in all cells, including nondividing cells, so we named them replication-independent EDSBs (RIND-EDSBs) [15]. RIND-EDSBs are located in hypermethylated DNA. Therefore, cells with global hypomethylation, such as cancer cells, have lower levels of RIND-EDSBs than noncancer cells [15]. After the discovery, we explored several characteristics of RIND-EDSBs and found that the majority of RIND-EDSBs possess physiological functions, namely, physiologic RIND-EDSBs (Phy-RIND-EDSBs), as epigenetic marks in maintaining genomic stability [16–19]. Interestingly, Phy-RIND-EDSBs in yeast decrease when yeast cells age [19]. So here I rename Phy-RIND-EDSBs in accordance with their role as youth-associated genomic-stabilizing DNA gaps (Youth-DNA-GAPs). In this chapter, we propose a hypothesis that the hypomethylated genome of the elderly reduces Phy-RIND-EDSBs and that this reduction causes DNA damage. The accumulation of DNA damage initiates DDR and consequently drives the cellular aging process (**Figure 1**).

In other words, the reduction in Phy-RIND-EDSBs by genome-wide hypomethylation is the underlying molecular pathogenesis mechanism of aging phenotypes.

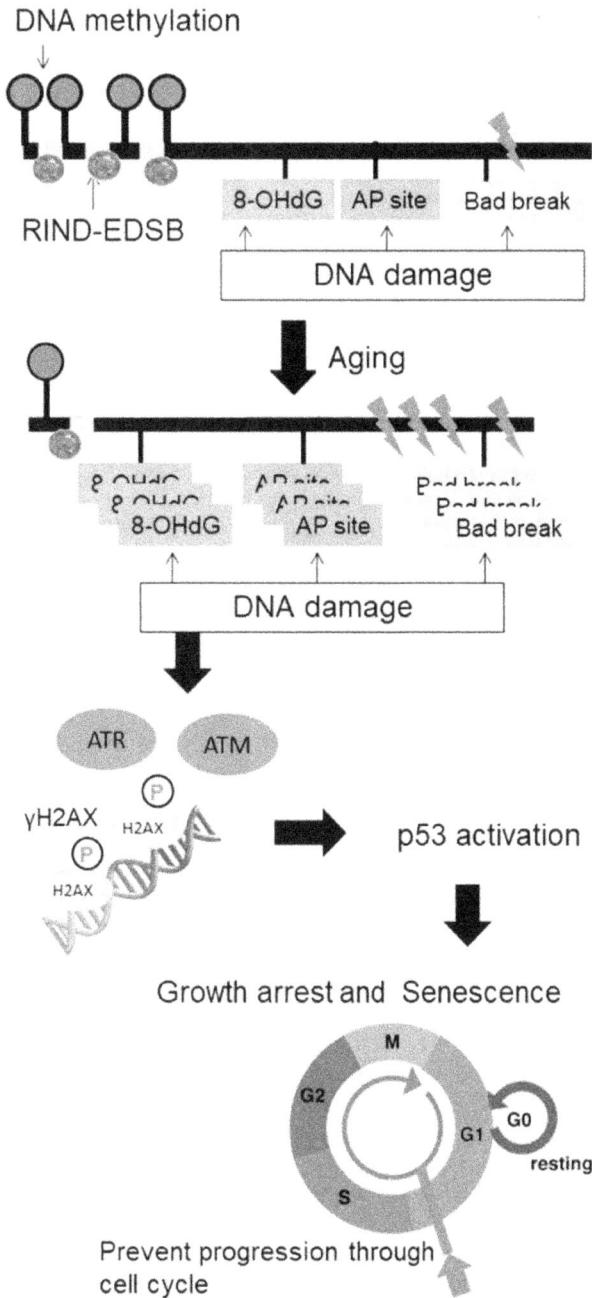

Figure 1.
Genome-wide hypomethylation drives genomic instability in the elderly by reducing youth-associated genome-stabilizing DNA gaps: A hypothesis. DNA methylation in the elderly is generally reduced, genome-wide hypomethylation. A reduction in DNA methylation leads to genomic instability, accumulation of endogenous DNA damage, and sensitivity to DNA-damaging agents. Here, we propose a hypothesis that global hypomethylation causes a reduction in Phy-RIND-EDSBs and that the reduction in Phy-RIND-EDSBs causes DNA damage. The accumulation of endogenous DNA damage will promote DDR, and too much DDR will arrest cells, causing metabolic rewiring and senescence.

2. Genome-wide hypomethylation

Genome-wide hypomethylation reduces the DNA methylation level of the whole genome. DNA methylation possesses two basic roles, gene regulation and the prevention of genomic instability, which we emphasize here [20]. The majority of DNA methylation in the human genome is on interspersed repetitive sequences (IRSs). Genome-wide hypomethylation or global hypomethylation mostly reflects a decrease in the DNA methylation of IRSs [11, 21]. Here, I will describe how IRS methylation occurs, how hypomethylation occurs, and how hypomethylation drives genomic instability in the elderly.

2.1 Interspersed repetitive sequence methylation

To evaluate the global methylation level, most recent studies have used PCR techniques to measure the DNA methylation level of each IRS, including Alu elements (Alu), long interspersed element-1s (LINE-1s), and several types of human endogenous retroviruses (HERVs). A reduction in Alu element methylation represents a genome-wide hypomethylation, driving genomic instability more than that of LINE-1 s and HERVs [11]. Throughout the human genome, there are over 1 million copies of Alu elements [22]. Although there is also a vast number of LINE-1 s, only approximately 3000 copies of LINE-1s contain a 5' UTR where LINE-1 methylation was usually measured [23, 24]. Because there are several classes of HERVs, each PCR measured DNA methylation of one class and as a result, covered a smaller percentage of the genome [25]. Furthermore, methylation of LINE-1 and HERV was reported to possess gene regulation functions [24, 26]. The tissue-specific methylation level of LINE-1 is locus dependent [27, 28]. In contrast, the global hypomethylation occurs as a generalized process [11, 28]. Therefore, methylation of LINE-1 and HERV represents global methylation in a lesser proportion than that of Alu elements.

2.2 Alu hypomethylation in aging and NCDs

Although global hypomethylation has been reported in the elderly, not all IRSs are hypomethylated. We investigated Alu, LINE-1, and HERV-K and found Alu and HERV-K hypomethylation in aging but not LINE-1 [11]. Therefore, methylation of LINE-1 and Alu may possess different roles. Global hypomethylation is also associated with the aging phenotype. First, lower global DNA methylation is associated with higher cardiovascular risk in postmenopausal women [29]. Second, Alu hypomethylation was observed in individuals with lower bone mass, osteopenia, osteoporosis, and a high body mass index [12]. Finally, Alu hypomethylation was reported in diabetes mellitus patients and was directly correlated with high fasting blood sugar, HbA1C, and blood pressure [13]. Interestingly, the Alu methylation level was also high in catch-up growth in a 20-year-old offspring [30]. These studies indicated the positive role of Alu methylation in the human growth process and the role of Alu hypomethylation as an epigenetic cause of the human aging process.

2.3 Mechanism causing global hypomethylation

The direct correlation between IRS methylation levels suggests that the mechanisms causing global hypomethylation in both aging cells and cancer are a generalizing process [11, 28]. The actual mechanism causing global hypomethylation in aging remains to be explored. Nevertheless, exposure to oxidative stress, benzene, air pollution, UV light, radiation, smoke, and folate deficiency facilitates genome-wide hypomethylation processes [31–37]. Therefore, the accumulation of

DNA damage, oxidative stress, or a lack of DNA methylation precursors can lead to genome-wide hypomethylation.

Evidence suggests that DNA damage drives the demethylation process. DNA repair, which is how cells remove DNA lesions, is also a demethylation mechanism that directly removes 5-methylcytosine. Methylcytosine is a DNA base that is prone to be deaminated and must be fixed by base excision repair (BER) machinery to prevent cytosine-to-thymine substitution. However, BER replaces the DNA lesion with an unmethylated form of cytosine. As a result, the methylcytosine is demethylated. The other mechanism is to remove the entire DNA patch and refill with unmethylated nucleotides by nucleotide excision repair (NER) or mismatch repair (MMR) [38].

For oxidative stress, oxidation of 5-methylcytosine forms 5-hydroxymethylcytosine. There are several mechanisms for removing 5-hydroxymethylcytosines and replacing them with unmethylated forms, AID/APOBEC enzymes and TET enzymes followed by BER [39–44]. Alternatively, oxidative stress may interfere with the DNA methylation protein machinery. For example, oxidative stress depletes the synthesis of glutathione and decreases the availability of S-adenosylmethionine for DNA methylation [45]. This proposed mechanism is similar to DNA demethylation in depletion of the methyl pool in folate-deficient models [46, 47].

2.4 Hypomethylation accumulates multiple kinds of DNA lesions

The hypomethylated genome is prone to accumulating multiple kinds of DNA damage, which is an abnormal chemical structure in DNA and includes oxidative damage, depurination, depyrimidination, and pathologic EDSBs [10, 14]. Alu methylation levels in white blood cells were found to inversely correlate with 8-hydroxy-2′-deoxyguanosine (8-OHdG) oxidative damage and apurinic/apyrimidinic sites (AP sites) [37]. Transfection of cells with Alu small interfering RNA (Alu siRNA) increased Alu methylation and reduced endogenous 8-OHdG and AP sites [37]. Interestingly, Alu siRNA also increased cell division and resistance to DNA damage-causing agents [37]. This evidence indirectly suggests that Alu methylation stabilizes the human genome. DNA methylation also prevents pathologic EDSBs. The chromosomal rearrangements and deletions of DNA commonly found in cancer cells treated with DNA demethylating agents and DNA methyltransferase (DNMT) knockout mice and naturally occurring mutations in the cytosine DNA methyltransferase DNMT3B suggest that pathologic EDSBs are the intermediate products of hypomethylation that drive genomic instability [10, 48–50].

2.5 DNA lesions as a molecular pathogenesis mechanism of the aging process and NCDs

A number of studies support the idea that accumulation of DNA damage drives the aging process. First, congenital defects in DNA repair accelerate aging. For example, progeroid syndrome patients with ERCC4 mutations have premature aging of many organs. ERCC4 is a protein designated as the DNA repair endonuclease XPF that is critical for many DNA repair pathways, including NER [51]. Second, genotoxic agents accelerate the aging process in cancer survivor patients. For example, 50-year-old survivors of childhood cancer have an increased incidence of age-related diseases compared to their siblings [52]. Third, there is evidence of DNA damage accumulation when cells age. Pathologic EDSBs are accumulated in chronological aging yeast [17]. Many kinds of DNA damage from base modifications to γH2AX foci, representing pathologic EDSBs, have been reported in several organs of animals and humans [53–56]. Finally, a reduction in DNA repair efficiency was reported in aging cells of many organisms [57–59]. In NCDs, the accumulation of oxidative DNA damage has been reported in patients with cardiovascular disease, diabetes and metabolic syndrome, chronic obstructive pulmonary disease, osteoporosis, and neurological degeneration, including Alzheimer's disease and Parkinson's disease [5]. DNA damage triggers DDR. To facilitate DNA repair and prevent mutation accumulation, DDR arrests cell cycle progression until repair is complete. While DDR can prevent cancer development, DDR leads to many unwanted effects, including inflammation, metabolic rewiring, senescence, apoptosis, and aging [60–62]. The DDR signaling pathway consists of signal sensors, transducers, and effectors. The sensors of this pathway are proteins that recognize DNA damage. The main transducers are ATM and ATR and their downstream kinases. The effectors of this pathway are substrates of ATM and ATR and their downstream kinases. These effectors of DDR involve many proteins, including P53, BRCA1, and CDC25s [60–63].

2.6 DNA methylation possesses a long-range effect in stabilizing the human genome in cis

A direct association between loss of DNA methylation and rearrangements in the pericentromeric heterochromatin was demonstrated in ICF syndrome (immunodeficiency, chromosomal instability, and facial anomalies) and loss-of-function mutations in DNMT3B [50, 64]. Therefore, hypomethylation could lead to spontaneous mutations in cis, which are epigenetic and genetic events occurring in the same chromosome. Notably, Alu siRNA increased Alu methylation levels in HEK293 cells from 60 to 70% [14]. Because there are approximately 1 million copies of Alu, by rough estimation, Alu siRNA methylates 10% of Alu elements or approximately 100,000 Alu elements in 3000 Mb of the human genome. In other words, Alu siRNA transfection methylated one locus of every 30 kb of human genome on average. Furthermore, Alu siRNA reduced 75% of endogenous 8-OHdG [14]. Therefore, even if Alu siRNA increases methylation in a limited location, the transfection stabilized the genome far beyond the methylated Alu elements (**Figure 2**).

2.7 Hypotheses: DNA methylation prevents genomic instability mechanisms

There are at least three possible mechanisms by which Alu methylation reduces endogenous DNA damage and increases resistance to DNA damage-causing agents. The extension of genomic stability from methylated Alu loci supports my first hypothesis that DNA methylation stabilizes the genome by homing Youth-DNA-GAPs, Phy-RIND-EDSBs, and that the gaps extended the stabilizing effect to the entire genome [14]. Another reason that supports the Phy-RIND-EDSBs mediating the DNA methylation role in stabilizing the genome is that Phy-RIND-EDSBs are localized in hypermethylated DNA [15]. Moreover, Phy-RIND-EDSBs possess a redundant topoisomerase which relieve tension of double-helix spin and torsion from any DNA activity [17]. The second hypothesis would be the spreading of DNA methylation and consequently heterochromatin [65]. However, this mechanism is unlikely because the spreading would need to extend to cover the whole genome and would interfere with cellular function. A reduction in cell viability by Alu siRNA was not observed. The last and unlikely hypothesis was that DNA methylation somehow enhanced DNA repair activity [66], although this mechanism is also unlikely because most DNA repair machinery starts with specific sensors to recognize DNA lesions.

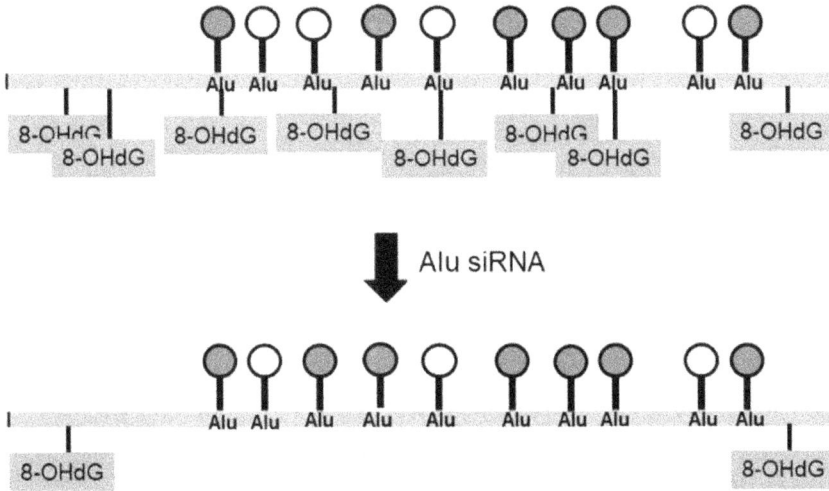

Figure 2.
DNA methylation possesses a long-range effect in stabilizing the human genome in cis. This diagram represents a fraction of the human genome before and after Alu siRNA transfection. While Alu siRNA methylated only 10% of Alu loci, Alu siRNA reduced 75% of the 8-OHdG in the entire genome [14]. Therefore, DNA methylation possesses a long-range effect in stabilizing the human genome. Blue circles are DNA methylation and white circles are unmethylated DNA.

3. Phy-RIND-EDSBs represent epigenetic marks as youth-DNA-GAPs

Phy-RIND-EDSBs are found in all eukaryotic cells, produced by certain proteins, and reduced in chronological aging yeast [15, 17, 19]. A reduction in Phy-RIND-EDSBs decreased cell viability and augmented pathologic EDSB production [19]. Phy-RIND-EDSBs are devoid of DDR and are repaired by the error-free repair pathway [16]. Therefore, Phy-RIND-EDSBs are Youth-DNA-GAPs epigenetic marks that prevent genomic instability in eukaryotic genomes.

3.1 IRS-EDSB ligation-mediated PCR (IRS-EDSB-LMPCR) to measure EDSBs

Ligation-mediated PCR (LMPCR) is the method that we used for EDSB detection [15]. Previously, this PCR technique was used to characterize the signal end and coding end of EDSBs occurring during the V(D)J recombination process [67]. For V(D)J recombination, the signal end and coding end of EDSBs occur at the T-cell receptor or antibody genes in lymphoblasts. To detect the signal end and coding end, DNA from lymphoblasts was ligated to a linker, and PCR was performed using linker primer and oligonucleotide sequences of T-cell receptor or antibody genes. Generalized EDSBs can occur anywhere in the genome. Therefore, we replaced IRS as a primer instead of T-cell receptor or antibody genes [67, 68]. As a result, IRS-EDSB-LMPCR yields two types of amplicons, IRS-EDSB and IRS-IRS sequences, and we detected linker sequences that represent EDSB amplicons. In brief, IRS-EDSB-LMPCR was performed as follows. First, the oligonucleotide linker, EDSB linker, was ligated to high-molecular-weight DNA (HMWDNA) or nucleus. Second, real-time quantitative PCR was performed using two PCR primers. The first was homologous to IRS, and the other had the same sequence as the 5′ end of the ligation linker. The number of EDSBs could be measured by Taqman probe homology to the 3′ end of the ligation linker sequence. The HMWDNA or nucleus served as a source of EDSBs, and the EDSB linker detected and ligated EDSBs. The first PCR cycle polymerized DNA from genome-wide distributed IRSs. The polymerization through EDSBs generated an EDSB-LMPCR linker template. The IRS-EDSB-linker sequences were generated, detected, and quantitated by the Taqman probe during PCR cycle (**Figure 3**) [15].

Common criticism of IRS-EDSB-LMPCR is the possibility of DNA shearing from HMWDNA preparation. However, the characteristics of the DSBs generated by DNA preparation are different from RIND-EDSBs. In humans, the sequence around RIND-EDSBs is always hypermethylated, whereas methylation levels of DSBs from mechanical shearing possess less methylation than RIND-EDSBs [15]. To prove that the RIND-EDSBs are real, we compared EDSBs from linker ligated to HMWDNA and nucleus and found that RIND-EDSBs analyzed directly from in situ ligation displayed the same pattern as IRS-EDSB-LMPCR from HMWDNA [17]. Therefore, DSBs detected by IRS-EDSB-LMPCR were endogenous in origin.

3.2 Phy-RIND-EDSBs are evolutionarily conserved epigenetic marks

Nature has conserved all epigenetic marks by conserving the genes that produce epigenetic marks [7]. Epigenetic marks have a specific biological role, whether it is gene expression, genomic stability, or interacting with DNA. Therefore, the genome distribution of epigenetic markers will not be random. Finally, epigenetic marks are usually crucial for cell survival and therefore should be ubiquitously present in all cells. To search for genes that produce or maintain Phy-RIND-EDSBs, we evaluated RIND-EDSB levels in yeast strains that lack functional mutation genes encoding various DNA repair regulators, chromatin formation, endonucleases, topoisomerase, and chromatin-condensing proteins [17]. We found low levels of RIND-EDSBs in cells lacking high-mobility group box (HMGB) proteins and Sir2. Thus, HMGB proteins and Sir2 play roles in producing and maintaining Phy-RIND-EDSBs [17]. Phy-RIND-EDSBs are distributed in the genome nonrandomly [18]. In humans, Phy-RIND-EDSBs are localized within hypermethylated DNA [15]. In yeast, DNA sequences 5′ end to RIND-EDSBs were not random; certain four-nucleotide sequences were more likely to be present immediately prior to the breaks. Moreover, RIND-EDSBs were prevented from occurring or were never observed following certain four-base combinations [18]. RIND-EDSBs were found in yeast and in the human genome, and therefore, Phy-RIND-EDSBs are conserved in eukaryotic organisms [15, 17]. In humans, RIND-EDSBs were detectable in all cell types and found within the hypermethylated genome in all phases of the cell cycle [15]. In yeast, we found a very strong direct correlation between cell viability and Phy-RIND-EDSB levels (r = 0.94, p < 0.0001) [19]. In other words, the more Phy-RIND-EDSBs a cell possesses, the better the cell survives [19]. When Phy-RIND-EDSB levels were reduced by homothallic switching (HO) endonuclease induction or NHP6A gene deletion, cell viability decreased [19]. In conclusion, Phy-RIND-EDSBs are epigenetic markers that are important in all eukaryotic cells [19].

Most of the RIND-EDSBs under normal physiologic conditions are not DNA damage, signals of the DDR, or precursors of mutations [16]. While sequences around human RIND-EDSBs are hypermethylated, γH2AX-binding DNA is hypomethylated. Therefore, most RIND-EDSBs are devoid of γH2AX [16]. γH2AX is a H2AX molecule that is phosphorylated at serine 139 by the signaling cascade of DDR of pathologic DSBs [69]. Most RIND-EDSBs are repaired by a more precise ATM-dependent pathway, and therefore, most RIND-EDSBs under normal physiologic conditions are Phy-RIND-EDSBs [16].

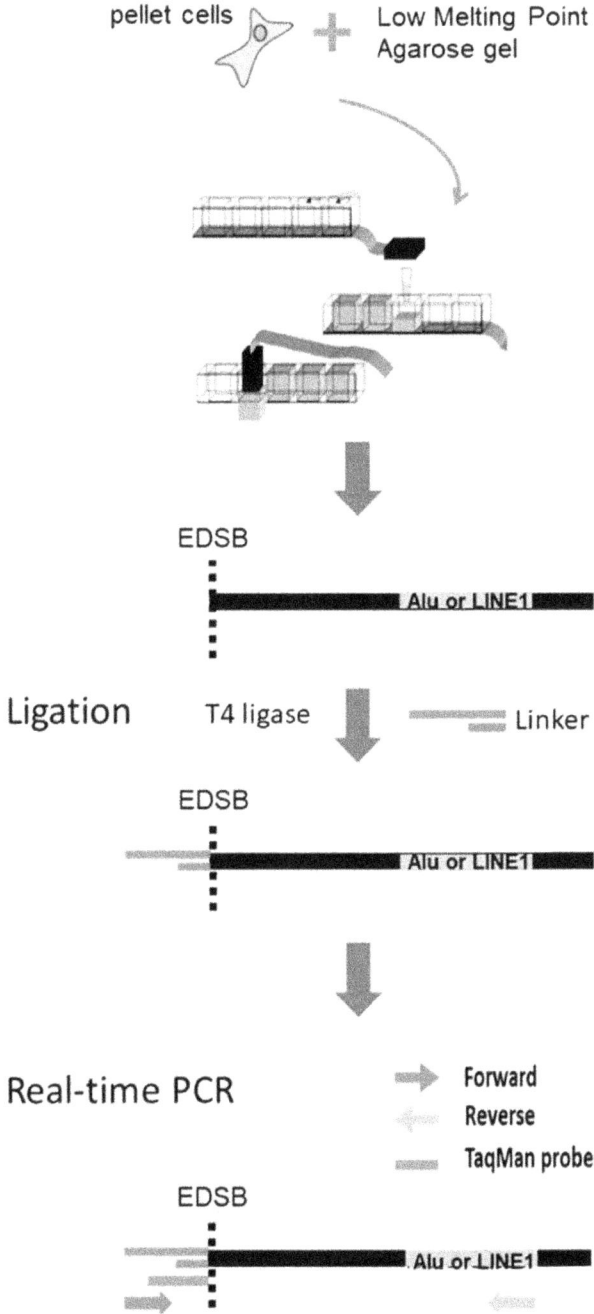

Figure 3.
IRS-EDSB-LMPCR diagram demonstrating IRS-EDSB-LMPCR. LMPCR linker ligates to EDSB. The 5' end of the LMPCR linker is the same sequence as the PCR primer. The 3' end of the LMPCR linker is homologous to the Taqman probe. The Taqman probe is used for quantitation of EDSBs by real-time PCR. The IRS primer is a PCR primer with IRS sequences to polymerize numerous locations of the genome [15].

3.3 Phy-RIND-EDSB or youth-DNA-GAP complex

Human Phy-RIND-EDSBs are localized in hypermethylated DNA regions and deacetylated histones [15, 16]. Phy-RIND-EDSBs are reduced in cells lacking HMGB proteins and Sir2 and NAD-dependent deacetylase [17, 70]. The human Sir2 homolog, sirtuin 1 (SIRT1), binds to the HMGB1 protein and deacetylates DNMT1 [71, 72]. Furthermore, HMGB1 possesses deoxyribophosphate lyase activity [73]. Therefore, we propose a hypothesis here that HMGB1 cuts DNA to produce Phy-RIND-EDSBs. SIRT1-bound HMGB1 deacetylates histones, keeping Phy-RIND-EDSB ends within the heterochromatin to shield them from the DDR signal. Finally, the interaction between SIRT1 and DNMT1 or deacetylated histone and DNA methylation may be the reason why sequences around human Phy-RIND-EDSBs are hypermethylated (**Figure 4**).

Interestingly, both HMGB1 and Sir2 have other functions that can be related to Phy-RIND-EDSBs. HMGB1 is a protein in another physiologic EDSB complex, the signal end and coding end of V(D)J recombination [74]. Moreover, yeast lacking the NHP6A protein, a type of yeast HMGB, shows increased endogenous DNA damage and sensitivity to UV light [75]. Finally, HMGB1 has the ability to bend DNA [76]. To prevent DNA torsion, it is reasonable to create Phy-RIND-EDSBs while bending DNA. Sir2 can deacetylate the histone, while Phy-RIND-EDSBs are localized in the deacetylated histone. Interestingly, Sir2 and SIRT1 are known to prevent the aging process [77, 78].

3.4 Spontaneous pathologic RIND-EDSBs and modified ends with insertion at the breaks

Independent of DNA replication, EDSB-LMPCR could detect pathologic RIND-EDSBs (Path-RIND-EDSBs) as excess EDSBs when DSB repair was inhibited by chemical inhibition or DSB repair gene mutation [19]. When we treated G0 yeast cells with caffeine, a DSB repair inhibitor, we observed a spontaneous increase in RIND-EDSBs [19]. These excess RIND-EDSBs did not possess the same 5′ end-sequence-four-base combinations as Phy-RIND-EDSBs odds ratio (OR) > 1 breaks. Notably, we called four-base combinations that are unlikely to be found in Phy-RIND-EDSBs as OR ≤ 1 breaks [18]. Moreover, we also observed that the 5′ end sequence downstream of the break did not match with the genomic sequence from the first base as reads with modified ends with insertion at the breaks (MIBs) [57]. We found that caffeine treatment increased the proportion

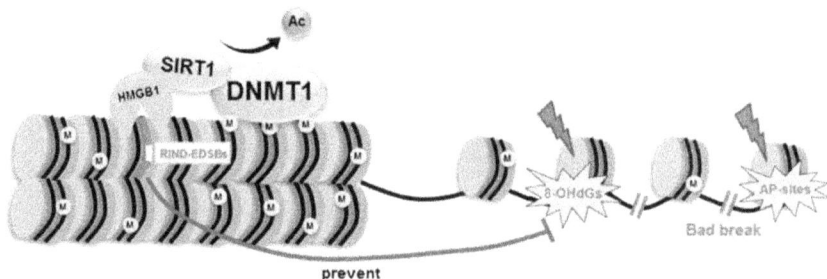

Figure 4.
Phy-RIND-EDSB or youth-DNA-GAP complex: I hypothesize that the HMGB group initiates Phy-RIND-EDSB and that HMGB interacts with SIR2 or SIRT1. SIRT1 deacetylates histones and DNMT1, and DNMT1 methylates DNA. The role of Phy-RIND-EDSB or youth-DNA-GAP is to prevent DNA damage anywhere along the same chromosome.

of MIBs [57]. Therefore, MIBs might be a mechanism that compensates for repair defects, such as alternate repair of the DSB pathway, or prevents EDSB ends from stimulating DDR. Seven repair defect yeast strains, *mec1Δ*, *mre11Δ*, *nej1Δ*, *rad51Δ*, *tel1Δ*, *yku70Δ*, and *yku80Δ*, were studied. Except for *nej1Δ*, the percentages of OR ≤ 1 breaks and MIBs were significantly increased in all samples when compared to the wild type. We also examined whether there was an association between MIBs and types of breaks (OR > 1 breaks and OR ≤ 1 breaks) and found that in the wild type, MIBs occurred at OR ≤ 1 breaks. In contrast, in *mec1Δ*, *mre11Δ*, *rad51Δ*, *tel1Δ*, *yku70Δ*, MIBs occurred at both OR > 1 breaks and OR ≤ 1 breaks [57]. Therefore, both Phy-RIND-EDSBs and Path-RIND-EDSBs are produced in the genome independent of DNA replication. However, most Path-RIND-EDSBs are immediately repaired, while Phy-RIND-EDSBs are retained [57].

3.5 Variation in RIND-EDSB level and reduction in Phy-RIND-EDSBs in aging and hypomethylated cells

Path-RIND-EDSBs are spontaneously produced and immediately repaired, while Phy-RIND-EDSBs are produced and retained by the Phy-RIND-EDSB complex formation process. We observed an increase in RIND-EDSB levels in yeast lacking a DSB repair gene, topoisomerase and endonuclease. Analysis of EDSB sequences suggested that DSB repair inhibition causes retention of both Phy-RIND-EDSBs and Path-RIND-EDSBs. For topoisomerase and endonuclease mutants, we postulated that Phy-RIND-EDSBs may have redundant roles with topoisomerase and endonuclease in stabilizing the genome. Nevertheless, sequence analysis is needed to prove this hypothesis. As mentioned earlier, one yeast strain lacking the *HMGB* gene or *SIR2* possessed a low level of RIND-EDSBs. Therefore, we hypothesized that HMGB and Sir2 play roles in PHY-RIND-EDSB complex formation and retention. We observed that three chemicals can alter RIND-EDSB levels. Whereas caffeine and vanillin, DSB repair inhibitors, increased RIND-EDSB levels, trichostatin A, a histone deacetylase inhibitor, decreased the EDSBs. The reduction in RIND-EDSBs by trichostatin A suggested that Phy-RIND-EDSBs are retained within facultative heterochromatin. This result is similar to the low level of RIND-EDSBs in yeast lacking *SIR2*.

DDR signals to repair Path-RIND-EDSBs can repair and consequently reduce Phy-RIND-EDSBs [19]. The retention of Phy-RIND-EDSBs and the immediate repair of Path-RIND-EDSBs led to the finding that the majority of RIND-EDSBs under normal physiologic conditions are Phy-RIND-EDSBs and that a reduction in RIND-EDSBs in any condition is a reduction in Phy-RIND-EDSBs. In addition to gene mutation and histone acetylation, we could reduce RIND-EDSB levels in yeast by inducing a Path-RIND-EDSB by HO endonuclease induction [19]. HO endonuclease is a site-specific endonuclease that cleaves a site in the MAT locus on chromosome III [79]. After induction in nondividing yeast, we observed a sustained reduction in RIND-EDSBs for up to 4 days. However, when we induced HO in yeast lacking *MEC1*, a DSB repair protein, the reduction was not observed [19]. These experiments suggested that Path-RIND-EDSB production can ignite the global DSB repair process, and consequently, the retained Phy-RIND-EDSBs are repaired [19]. This mechanism is one possible explanation for the reduction in RIND-EDSBs in chronologically aging yeast.

Phy-RIND-EDSB levels in the elderly should be low. We found low levels of RIND-EDSBs in chronologically aging yeast and in the human cancer cells, HeLa and SW480, which are cervical cancer and colon cancer cell lines, respectively [15, 19]. Phy-RIND-EDSBs are localized in hypermethylated genomic regions [15].

Therefore, cancer genome hypomethylation may explain why RIND-EDSB levels in cancer cells were low [15, 27]. We have not reported RIND-EDSB levels in the elderly. However, our unpublished data demonstrated results similar to those in chronologically aging yeast and in cancer cells.

3.6 Reduction in Phy-RIND-EDSBs augments pathologic EDSB production

To define the molecular mechanism by which the reduction in Phy-RIND-EDSBs in chronological aging in yeast reduced cell viability and to evaluate the consequences of Phy-RIND-EDSB reduction, we analyzed yeast cells with low levels of Phy-RIND-EDSBs, including HO endonuclease and *nhp6aΔ*, a high-mobility group box protein mutant [19]. Very high levels of Path-RIND-EDSBs were observed in both strains possessing low levels of Phy-RIND-EDSBs after treatment with caffeine, a DSB repair inhibitor. The new Path-RIND-EDSBs were not in the same location as Phy-RIND-EDSBs. Therefore, similar to DNA methylation, Phy-RIND-EDSB stabilizes the genome far beyond the Phy-RIND-EDSB complex (**Figure 4**). These experiments led to my conclusion that the role of Phy-RIND-EDSBs is similar to that of EDSBs induced by topoisomerase, which is DNA torsion prevention and DNA tension reduction from DNA spinning due to any DNA activity, including transcription, replication, and repair. The role of Phy-RIND-EDSBs can be imagined as gaps in a railroad track that prevent track torsion from track expansion by heat. Phy-RIND-EDSB levels decreased in chronologically aging yeast, and the reduction was directly correlated with reduced cell viability. Therefore, Phy-RIND-EDSBs play a Youth-DNA-GAPs role in preventing Path-RIND-EDSBs and DNA damage lesions [19]. Moreover, the *nhp6a* gene is known to prevent other types of DNA lesions, such as pyrimidine dimers [75]. Therefore, it is reasonable to hypothesize that the scatter distribution of the Phy-RIND-EDSB complex prevents all kinds of DNA damage along the length of the whole genome (**Figure 4**).

3.7 DNA repair activity may be compromised in aging cells by a reduction in Phy-RIND-EDSBs

A reduction in Phy-RIND-EDSBs during chronological aging may be a cause of DNA repair defects in the elderly. DNA repair machinery is known to be compromised and error-prone with age [59, 75]. Numerous studies have found a significant decline in all commonly known repair pathway activities with aging, including double-strand break repair activities [53–56]. We demonstrated that the reduction in the Phy-RIND-EDSB complex will increase the production of DNA damage [19]. Therefore, aging cells have to repair DNA damage more often than younger cells. As a result, more DNA repair machinery is required for older cells. Consequently, DNA repair substrates are consumed more quickly than they are produced, resulting in DNA repair defects in the elderly.

4. Conclusion

All evidences described in this chapter suggest that genomic instability in the elderly is a vicious cycle of interactive networks among DNA damage, DNA repair, DNA demethylation, and reduction in Youth-DNA-GAPs (**Figure 5**). DNA damage occurs spontaneously. Then, the DNA repair process, in addition to repairing DNA damage, has consequences of reducing epigenetic marks. While NER demethylates DNA, the DSB repair pathway will repair Phy-RIND-EDSBs. DNA demethylation

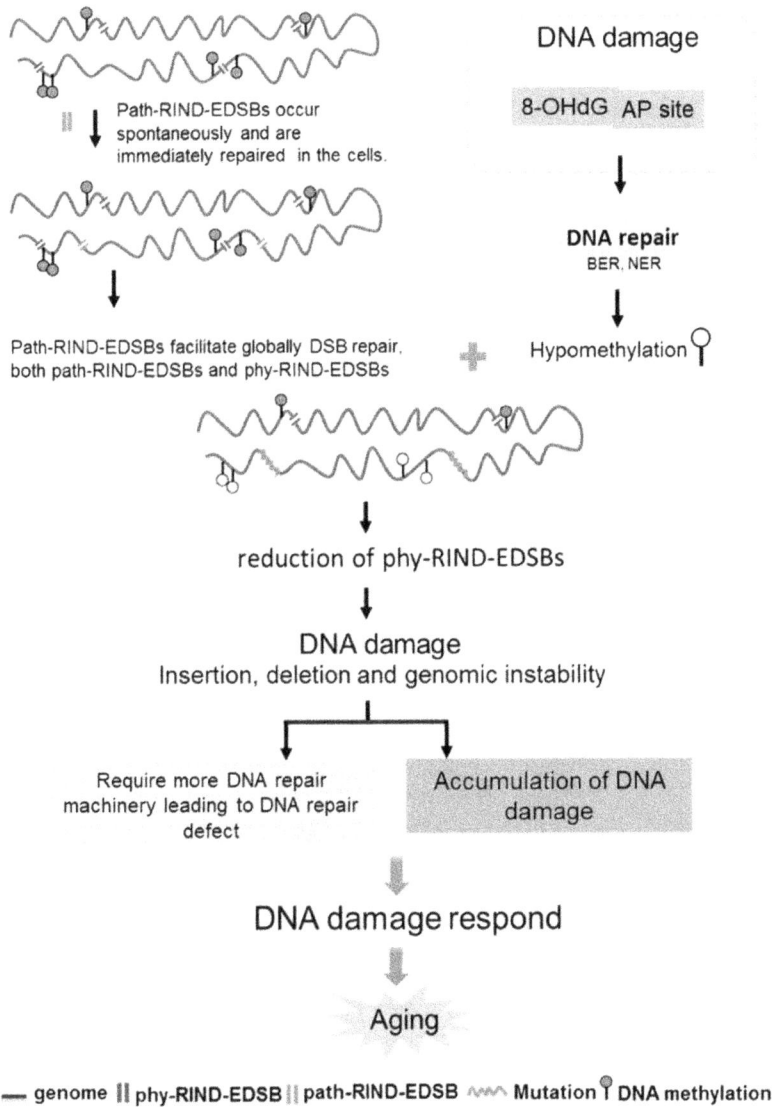

Figure 5.
Destructive network of aging DNA. DNA damage can occur spontaneously. The base modification repair consequence is DNA demethylation, and DSB repair for pathologic DSB will also globally repair Phy-RIND-EDSBs. Continuous DNA demethylation results in genome-wide hypomethylation, which, together with global Phy-RIND-EDSB repair, reduces the Phy-RIND-EDSB complex. A reduction in the Phy-RIND-EDSB complex augments DNA damage, and a large amount of DNA damage requires extensive DDR. Cells extensively use DDR until the DNA repair machinery is exhausted and defective, at which point, DNA damage accumulates and DDR arrests and ages cells.

results in global hypomethylation and consequently reduces the homing of Phy-RIND-EDSBs. The depletion of the Phy-RIND-EDSB complex will then augment DNA damage production. Cells need to use many DNA repair substrates to eliminate DNA damage faster than these substrates are produced and eventually lose the capability of DNA repair. As a result, aging cells continue to accumulate DNA damage and send DDR signals, halting the cell cycle, causing metabolic rewiring, and eventually driving cells to enter senescence.

Acknowledgements

All studies in Thailand were supported by the National Science and Technology Development Agency, Thailand Research Fund, and Chulalongkorn University, Thailand. I thank Dr. Maturada Patchsung, Ms Papitchaya Watcharanurak, and Ms. Sirapat Settayanon for illustration design.

Conflict of interest

The author declares no conflict of interest.

Abbreviation list

NCDs	noncommunicable disease
DDR	DNA damage repair signal
EDSB	endogenous DNA double-strand break
RIND-EDSB	replication-independent endogenous DNA double-strand break
Phy-RIND-EDSBs	physiologic RIND-EDSBs
Youth-DNA-GAPs	youth-associated genomic-stabilizing DNA gaps
IRSs	interspersed repetitive sequences
Alu	Alu elements
LINE-1s	long interspersed element-1s
HERVs	human endogenous retroviruses
BER	base excision repair
NER	nucleotide excision repair
MMR	mismatch repair
8-OHdG	8-hydroxy-2′-deoxyguanosine
AP sites	apurinic/apyrimidinic sites
DNMT	DNA methyltransferase
Alu siRNA	Alu small interfering RNA
LMPCR	ligation-mediated PCR
HMW DNA	high-molecular-weight DNA
IRS-EDSB-LMPCR	IRS-EDSB ligation-mediated PCR
HMGB	high-mobility group box
SIRT1	sirtuin 1
Path-RIND-EDSBs	pathologic RIND-EDSBs
HO	homothallic switching
OR	odds ratio
MIBs	modified ends with insertion at the breaks

Author details

Apiwat Mutirangura
Department of Anatomy, Faculty of Medicine, Institution(s), Center for Excellence
in Molecular Genetics of Cancer and Human Diseases, Chulalongkorn University,
Bangkok, Thailand

*Address all correspondence to: mapiwat@chula.ac.th
and apiwat.mutirangura@gmail.com

IntechOpen

References

[1] Lopez-Otin C et al. The hallmarks of aging. Cell. 2013;**153**(6):1194-1217

[2] Hanahan D, Weinberg RA. Hallmarks of cancer: The next generation. Cell. 2011;**144**(5):646-674

[3] Schumacher B, Garinis GA, Hoeijmakers JH. Age to survive: DNA damage and aging. Trends in Genetics. 2008;**24**(2):77-85

[4] Olivieri F et al. DNA damage response (DDR) and senescence: Shuttled inflamma-miRNAs on the stage of inflamm-aging. Oncotarget. 2015;**6**(34):35509-35521

[5] Milic M et al. DNA damage in non-communicable diseases: A clinical and epidemiological perspective. Mutation Research. 2015;**776**:118-127

[6] Huang B, Jiang C, Zhang R. Epigenetics: The language of the cell? Epigenomics. 2014;**6**(1):73-88

[7] Mazzio EA, Soliman KF. Basic concepts of epigenetics: Impact of environmental signals on gene expression. Epigenetics. 2012;**7**(2):119-130

[8] De Bont R, van Larebeke N. Endogenous DNA damage in humans: A review of quantitative data. Mutagenesis. 2004;**19**(3):169-185

[9] Unnikrishnan A et al. Revisiting the genomic hypomethylation hypothesis of aging. Annals of the New York Academy of Sciences. 2018;**1418**(1):69-79

[10] Chen RZ et al. DNA hypomethylation leads to elevated mutation rates. Nature. 1998;**395**(6697):89-93

[11] Jintaridth P, Mutirangura A. Distinctive patterns of age-dependent hypomethylation in interspersed repetitive sequences. Physiological Genomics. 2010;**41**(2):194-200

[12] Jintaridth P et al. Hypomethylation of Alu elements in post-menopausal women with osteoporosis. PLoS One. 2013;**8**(8):e70386

[13] Thongsroy J, Patchsung M, Mutirangura A. The association between Alu hypomethylation and severity of type 2 diabetes mellitus. Clinical Epigenetics. 2017;**9**:93

[14] Patchsung M et al. Alu siRNA to increase Alu element methylation and prevent DNA damage. Epigenomics. 2018;**10**(2):175-185

[15] Pornthanakasem W et al. LINE-1 methylation status of endogenous DNA double-strand breaks. Nucleic Acids Research. 2008;**36**(11):3667-3675

[16] Kongruttanachok N et al. Replication independent DNA double-strand break retention may prevent genomic instability. Molecular Cancer. 2010;**9**:70

[17] Thongsroy J et al. Replication-independent endogenous DNA double-strand breaks in *Saccharomyces cerevisiae* model. PLoS One. 2013;**8**(8):e72706

[18] Pongpanich M et al. Characteristics of replication-independent endogenous double-strand breaks in *Saccharomyces cerevisiae*. BMC Genomics. 2014;**15**:750

[19] Thongsroy J et al. Reduction in replication-independent endogenous DNA double-strand breaks promotes genomic instability during chronological aging in yeast. The FASEB Journal. 2018:fj201800218RR

[20] Tirado-Magallanes R et al. Whole genome DNA methylation: Beyond genes silencing. Oncotarget. 2017;**8**(3):5629-5637

[21] Zheng Y et al. Prediction of genome-wide DNA methylation in repetitive elements. Nucleic Acids Research. 2017;**45**(15):8697-8711

[22] International Human Genome Sequencing Consortium. Finishing the euchromatic sequence of the human genome. Nature. 2004;**431**(7011):931-945

[23] Penzkofer T et al. L1Base 2: More retrotransposition-active LINE-1s, more mammalian genomes. Nucleic Acids Research. 2017;**45**(D1):D68-D73

[24] Aporntewan C et al. Hypomethylation of intragenic LINE-1 represses transcription in cancer cells through AGO2. PLoS One. 2011;**6**(3):e17934

[25] Gifford RJ et al. Nomenclature for endogenous retrovirus (ERV) loci. Retrovirology. 2018;**15**(1):59

[26] Tongyoo P et al. EnHERV: Enrichment analysis of specific human endogenous retrovirus patterns and their neighboring genes. PLoS One. 2017;**12**(5):e0177119

[27] Chalitchagorn K et al. Distinctive pattern of LINE-1 methylation level in normal tissues and the association with carcinogenesis. Oncogene. 2004;**23**(54):8841-8846

[28] Phokaew C et al. LINE-1 methylation patterns of different loci in normal and cancerous cells. Nucleic Acids Research. 2008;**36**(17):5704-5712

[29] Ramos RB et al. Association between global leukocyte DNA methylation and cardiovascular risk in postmenopausal women. BMC Medical Genetics. 2016;**17**(1):71

[30] Rerkasem K et al. Higher Alu methylation levels in catch-up growth in twenty-year-old offsprings. PLoS One. 2015;**10**(3):e0120032

[31] Bollati V et al. Changes in DNA methylation patterns in subjects exposed to low-dose benzene. Cancer Research. 2007;**67**(3):876-880

[32] Mittal A et al. Exceptionally high protection of photocarcinogenesis by topical application of (−-)-epigallocatechin-3-gallate in hydrophilic cream in SKH-1 hairless mouse model: Relationship to inhibition of UVB-induced global DNA hypomethylation. Neoplasia. 2003;**5**(6):555-565

[33] Koturbash I et al. Radiation-induced changes in DNA methylation of repetitive elements in the mouse heart. Mutation Research. 2016;**787**:43-53

[34] Puttipanyalears C et al. Alu hypomethylation in smoke-exposed epithelia and oral squamous carcinoma. Asian Pacific Journal of Cancer Prevention. 2013;**14**(9):5495-5501

[35] Wangsri S et al. Patterns and possible roles of LINE-1 methylation changes in smoke-exposed epithelia. PLoS One. 2012;**7**(9):e45292

[36] Crider KS et al. Folate and DNA methylation: A review of molecular mechanisms and the evidence for folate's role. Advances in Nutrition. 2012;**3**(1):21-38

[37] Patchsung M et al. Long interspersed nuclear element-1 hypomethylation and oxidative stress: Correlation and bladder cancer diagnostic potential. PLoS One. 2012;**7**(5):e37009

[38] Grin I, Ishchenko AA. An interplay of the base excision repair and mismatch repair pathways in active DNA demethylation. Nucleic Acids Research. 2016;**44**(8):3713-3727

[39] Wu SC, Zhang Y. Active DNA demethylation: Many roads lead to Rome. Nature Reviews. Molecular Cell Biology. 2010;**11**(9):607-620

[40] Globisch D et al. Tissue distribution of 5-hydroxymethylcytosine and search for active demethylation intermediates. PLoS One. 2010;**5**(12):e15367

[41] Guo JU et al. Hydroxylation of 5-methylcytosine by TET1 promotes active DNA demethylation in the adult brain. Cell. 2011;**145**(3):423-434

[42] Pfaffeneder T et al. The discovery of 5-formylcytosine in embryonic stem cell DNA. Angewandte Chemie (International Ed. in English). 2011;**50**(31):7008-7012

[43] He YF et al. Tet-mediated formation of 5-carboxylcytosine and its excision by TDG in mammalian DNA. Science. 2011;**333**(6047):1303-1307

[44] Ito S et al. Tet proteins can convert 5-methylcytosine to 5-formylcytosine and 5-carboxylcytosine. Science. 2011;**333**(6047):1300-1303

[45] Hitchler MJ, Domann FE. An epigenetic perspective on the free radical theory of development. Free Radical Biology & Medicine. 2007;**43**(7):1023-1036

[46] Miller JW et al. Folate-deficiency-induced homocysteinaemia in rats: Disruption of S-adenosylmethionine's coordinate regulation of homocysteine metabolism. The Biochemical Journal. 1994;**298**(Pt 2):415-419

[47] Miller JW et al. Folate, DNA methylation, and mouse models of breast tumorigenesis. Nutrition Reviews. 2008;**66**(Suppl 1):S59-S64

[48] Eden A et al. Chromosomal instability and tumors promoted by DNA hypomethylation. Science. 2003;**300**(5618):455

[49] Lengauer C, Kinzler KW, Vogelstein B. DNA methylation and genetic instability in colorectal cancer cells. Proceedings of the National Academy of Sciences of the United States of America. 1997;**94**(6):2545-2550

[50] Xu GL et al. Chromosome instability and immunodeficiency syndrome caused by mutations in a DNA methyltransferase gene. Nature. 1999;**402**(6758):187-191

[51] Niedernhofer LJ et al. A new progeroid syndrome reveals that genotoxic stress suppresses the somatotroph axis. Nature. 2006;**444**(7122):1038-1043

[52] Armstrong GT et al. Aging and risk of severe, disabling, life-threatening, and fatal events in the childhood cancer survivor study. Journal of Clinical Oncology. 2014;**32**(12):1218-1227

[53] Siddiqui MS et al. Persistent gammaH2AX: A promising molecular marker of DNA damage and aging. Mutation Research, Reviews in Mutation Research. 2015;**766**:1-19

[54] Voss P, Siems W. Clinical oxidation parameters of aging. Free Radical Research. 2006;**40**(12):1339-1349

[55] Poljsak B, Dahmane R. Free radicals and extrinsic skin aging. Dermatology Research and Practice. 2012;**2012**:135206

[56] Al-Mashhadi S et al. Oxidative glial cell damage associated with white matter lesions in the aging human brain. Brain Pathology. 2015;**25**(5):565-574

[57] Pongpanich M, Patchsung M, Mutirangura A. Pathologic replication-independent endogenous DNA double-Strand breaks repair defect in chronological aging yeast. Frontiers in Genetics. 2018;**9**:501

[58] Gorbunova V et al. Changes in DNA repair during aging. Nucleic Acids Research. 2007;**35**(22):7466-7474

[59] Li W, Vijg J. Measuring genome instability in aging—A mini-review. Gerontology. 2012;**58**(2):129-138

[60] Ciccia A, Elledge SJ. The DNA damage response: Making it safe to play with knives. Molecular Cell. 2010;**40**(2):179-204

[61] Harper JW, Elledge SJ. The DNA damage response: Ten years after. Molecular Cell. 2007;**28**(5):739-745

[62] Turgeon MO, Perry NJS, Poulogiannis G. DNA damage, repair, and cancer metabolism. Frontiers in Oncology. 2018;**8**:15

[63] Marechal A, Zou L. DNA damage sensing by the ATM and ATR kinases. Cold Spring Harbor Perspectives in Biology. 2013:**5**(9)

[64] Qu GZ et al. Frequent hypomethylation in Wilms tumors of DNA in chromosomes 1 and 16. Cancer Genetics and Cytogenetics, 1999. **109**(1): p. 34-39

[65] Meng H et al. DNA methylation, its mediators and genome integrity. International Journal of Biological Sciences. 2015;**11**(5):604-617

[66] Putiri EL, Robertson KD. Epigenetic mechanisms and genome stability. Clinical Epigenetics. 2011;**2**(2):299-314

[67] Steen SB et al. Initiation of V(D)J recombination in vivo: Role of recombination signal sequences in formation of single and paired double-strand breaks. The EMBO Journal. 1997;**16**(10):2656-2664

[68] Schlissel MS. Structure of nonhairpin coding-end DNA breaks in cells undergoing V(D)J recombination. Molecular and Cellular Biology. 1998;**18**(4):2029-2037

[69] Kuo LJ, Yang LX. Gamma-H2AX—A novel biomarker for DNA double-strand breaks. In Vivo. 2008;**22**(3):305-309

[70] Shore D. The Sir2 protein family: A novel deacetylase for gene silencing and more. Proceedings of the National Academy of Sciences of the United States of America. 2000;**97**(26):14030-14032

[71] Hwang JS et al. Deacetylation-mediated interaction of SIRT1-HMGB1 improves survival in a mouse model of endotoxemia. Scientific Reports. 2015;**5**:15971

[72] Peng L et al. SIRT1 deacetylates the DNA methyltransferase 1 (DNMT1) protein and alters its activities. Molecular and Cellular Biology. 2011;**31**(23):4720-4734

[73] Prasad R et al. HMGB1 is a cofactor in mammalian base excision repair. Molecular Cell. 2007;**27**(5):829-841

[74] Ru H et al. Molecular mechanism of V(D)J recombination from synaptic RAG1-RAG2 complex structures. Cell. 2015;**163**(5):1138-1152

[75] Giavara S et al. Yeast Nhp6A/B and mammalian Hmgb1 facilitate the maintenance of genome stability. Current Biology. 2005;**15**(1):68-72

[76] Stros M. HMGB proteins: Interactions with DNA and chromatin. Biochimica et Biophysica Acta. 2010;**1799**(1-2):101-113

[77] Poulose N, Raju R. Sirtuin regulation in aging and injury. Biochimica et Biophysica Acta. 2015;**1852**(11):2442-2455

[78] Wierman MB, Smith JS. Yeast sirtuins and the regulation of aging. FEMS Yeast Research. 2014;**14**(1):73-88

[79] Nasmyth K. Regulating the HO endonuclease in yeast. Current Opinion in Genetics & Development. 1993;**3**(2):286-294

www.ingramcontent.com/pod-product-compliance
Lightning Source LLC
Chambersburg PA
CBHW081236190326
41458CB00016B/5802